FROM LOSS TO MEMORY

How do the billions of connections between neurons in our brain change as we learn and remember? This is the story of the discovery and the discoverer of synaptic pruning, the process of synapse elimination central to making us who we are. Through Professor Peter Huttenlocher's childhood in wartime and post-war Germany, his emigration to the US to reunite with his mother, and the launch and progressive stages of a career in medicine and research, the motivations and process of scientific discovery that led to an unexpected leap in our understanding of the human brain are uncovered. Accessible examples illustrate how, decades later, researchers are discovering the importance of synaptic pruning in early learning, autism, schizophrenia and Alzheimer's disease.

Physician scientist Anna Huttenlocher is a Professor at University of Wisconsin, Madison and a member of the National Academy of Medicine. Her laboratory studies cell migration in inflammation and cancer. She directed the MD-Ph.D. program at UW-Madison and is a committed mentor to the next generation of physicians and biomedical scientists.

From Loss to Memory

Behind the Discovery of Synaptic Pruning

ANNA HUTTENLOCHER
University of Wisconsin, Madison

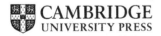
CAMBRIDGE
UNIVERSITY PRESS

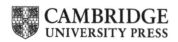

Shaftesbury Road, Cambridge CB2 8EA, United Kingdom

One Liberty Plaza, 20th Floor, New York, NY 10006, USA

477 Williamstown Road, Port Melbourne, VIC 3207, Australia

314–321, 3rd Floor, Plot 3, Splendor Forum, Jasola District Centre, New Delhi – 110025, India

103 Penang Road, #05–06/07, Visioncrest Commercial, Singapore 238467

Cambridge University Press is part of Cambridge University Press & Assessment, a department of the University of Cambridge.

We share the University's mission to contribute to society through the pursuit of education, learning and research at the highest international levels of excellence.

www.cambridge.org
Information on this title: www.cambridge.org/9781009267069

DOI: 10.1017/9781009267038

First published 2023
First paperback edition 2024

A catalogue record for this publication is available from the British Library

Library of Congress Cataloging-in-Publication data
Names: Huttenlocher, Anna, author.
Title: From loss to memory : behind the discovery of synaptic pruning / Anna Huttenlocher.
Description: Cambridge, United Kingdom ; New York, NY : Cambridge University Press, 2023. | Includes bibliographical references and index.
Identifiers: LCCN 2023000666 | ISBN 9781009267052 (hardback) | ISBN 9781009267069 (paperback) | ISBN 9781009267038 (ebook)
Subjects: MESH: Huttenlocher, Peter R. | Physicians | Neurologists | Neuronal Plasticity | Emigrants and Immigrants | Germany | United States | Biography
Classification: LCC R690 | NLM WZ 100 | DDC 610.92 [B]–dc23/eng/20230317
LC record available at https://lccn.loc.gov/2023000666

ISBN   978-1-009-26705-2   Hardback
ISBN   978-1-009-26706-9   Paperback

....

For Peter

CONTENTS

PREFACE

This book is the story of the life of Peter Huttenlocher, the pediatric neurologist and physician scientist who discovered synaptic pruning. The book carries interlaced themes – provocative examples of the career path of a physician scientist and the process of scientific discovery, discussion of a surprisingly broad set of social and medical fields that are being impacted by our knowledge of synaptic pruning and a biography of a child of wartime Germany who emerged, through complex twists and turns, to live an engaging life.

I write this book from the perspective of a physician scientist, but also as Peter Huttenlocher's daughter. I would like to acknowledge this inherent bias. Many objective sources were utilized to provide balance in this presentation of Peter Huttenlocher's life and work. The letters and other documents are from Peter Huttenlocher's personal collection. Many of the letters and other documents are translated from German. Other sources include published documents, personal conversations and interviews with neuroscientists and neurologists.

The idea to write this book arose after I attended a conference in Sicily in 2016. My own research focuses on the cell biology of inflammation. The conference was entitled "A Hundred Years of the Phagocyte," in recognition of the "father" of innate immunity, Elie Metchnikoff. At this meeting I was startled to see a slide from my father's 1979 paper first describing synaptic pruning. Professor Beth Stevens (Harvard Medical School) discussed his work as a key inspiration for her subsequent work focused on microglial cells and synaptic pruning. After her talk my puzzled colleagues asked: was that your work on synapses? My response: "Umm … I was a kid when that work was done – by my father." It is unusual to see decades-old figures presented at current-day scientific conferences. This tends to be done only for truly ground-breaking studies. It made me realize the long-lasting impact of my father's work, and how the significance of these findings had only gained broader recognition in the final years of his life and after his passing. Seeing the work on synaptic pruning presented at a conference 35 years after it was first published – and subsequently learning that his figures are often shown at neuroscience conferences – provided the motivation for writing this book about my father's life and work.

Peter was driven throughout his career to understand how the human brain develops in health and disease. A witness to human atrocity during his childhood in wartime Germany, he also was intrigued by the way the environment influences the development of the human brain during childhood. He took on the old question of "nature versus nurture" during brain development. This question became a particular focus for Peter later in his career, at the end of which he wrote a book entitled *Neural Plasticity: The Effects of Environment on the Development of the Cerebral Cortex* (Harvard University Press, 2002). This is particularly interesting because, throughout much of his life, he hid his own painful childhood memories, even as he worked to understand how the human brain develops and discovered a process, synapse elimination, that is central to the formation of human memory.

The present book is written to make the science accessible. The fields of synapse biology and cognitive neuroscience are broad and exhaustive. The book has been written for a wide-ranging audience and focused on only certain aspects of the field of synaptic pruning, such as recent developments in the area of microglia-mediated synapse elimination. There are multiple exciting areas of neuroscience, which I do not cover, that have significant relevance to synaptic pruning. These include rapid progress in understanding the cell biology of the synapse, the biology of astrocytes, the chemistry of synaptic transmission and work related to synaptic potentiation and depression critical for the formation of human memories. Relevant topics regarding the role of synaptic pruning in medical neurology, psychiatry, psychology and education are discussed. However, the scope of these fields is vast, with many additional areas of rapid and exciting discovery.

My hope is that this telling will be understandable for the student, scientist, physician, psychologist and any persons interested in German history, medicine or science more broadly. This book interweaves science and history to provide insight into the career of a unique pediatric neurologist and cognitive neuroscientist. A number of chapters explore where the discovery of synaptic pruning has taken us four decades later. More centrally, the book tells of the discoverer: the uncommon route through which a child grew into a physician scientist and followed his curiosity to understand the human brain. It is the story of a physician and scientist who, between seeing patients, "dabbled" in the laboratory and, more than once, made fundamental discoveries about how the human brain works.

ACKNOWLEDGMENTS

This book would not have been possible without the support, encouragement and critical reading by my husband, Andrew Bent. I would like to acknowledge the following people for help with translations: Ruth Altman, Marion Hofmann Bowman and Ludwig Decke. I would also like to thank the following people for critical reading: Jason Bent, Mina Bakhtiar, Margaret Plank and Yevgenya Grinblat. Finally, I would like to thank the scientists and family members who provided many useful discussions and interviews that form the basis of this book. In particular, I would like to acknowledge my father Peter and my uncle Wolfgang for the detailed descriptions of their lives in Germany, both during and after the war.

1 COUNTING SYNAPSES

My father, a practicing pediatric neurologist, was also a scientist. As a child, I remember my father peering at hundreds of micrographs of neuronal connections. Billions of these small connections form between neurons in the developing brain. Over the years he counted many, many synapses in post-mortem brain samples. A US immigrant who grew up in wartime Germany, he quietly shouldered his own childhood experiences. And he gained lasting fame – among neuroscientists and others – by discovering something fundamental. Brain synaptic connections increase dramatically during early human development, as anyone might expect. But Peter – Dad – Dr. Huttenlocher – discovered that, by the millions, these connections are also selectively removed as we learn and develop. This process, now referred to as synaptic pruning, is the process of refinement that mediates our skills, our abilities and our memories [1].

Peter was born in Oberlahnstein bei Koblenz, in Germany, in 1931 (Figure 1.1). He was the younger of two brothers born to Else, an opera singer, and Richard, a chemist. Peter remembered being the *Dümmling* ("simpleton") in the family. He was often distracted and struggled in school as a young child. Peter adored his mother. He and his brother Dieter would run along cobbled streets to the train station to greet their mother when she returned from work singing in the Cologne opera. Peter had few other memories from his young childhood with his mother, before she fled Germany in 1936.

The details of what happened only emerged gradually. In a brief first telling, Else had visibility as a dramatic soprano in the Cologne Opera. But she refused to join the state-mandated music guild, the *Reichmusikkammer*, and this drew the attention of the authorities and endangered her family. Her legendarily strong and proud demeanor included elements of being stubborn and this included being stubbornly supportive of her artist/musician friends and colleagues who were Jewish. The months passed. The Nazi movement deepened its inroads into lives and communities. Else was banned from singing and her passport was confiscated. With little public notice, but nonetheless noticeably, "undesirable" persons were being taken from their homes. Else and Richard divorced. The *Fürsorge* (child welfare) authorities declared that Else was

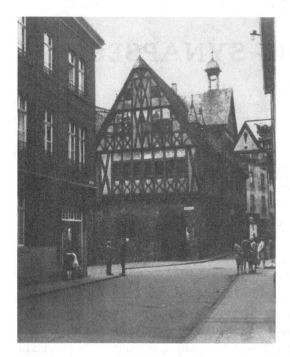

Figure 1.1 The streets of Oberlahnstein in 1930 shortly before Peter's birth.

expressly unable to raise "Aryan children," and Richard was given full custody of young Dieter and Peter. After Else shamed the authorities about honoring a prior commitment to sing at a Belgian opera house, her passport was temporarily returned and she was allowed passage by the Nazis, only for this single performance. She did not return. From Belgium, Else later received safe passage and sponsorship to travel to the United States. While Else lived in Belgium, and later France, Peter and Dieter traveled by train, with their father, to visit their mother. A photograph shows Peter, six years old, with his mother and Dieter in Spa, Belgium, near the train station (Figure 1.2). The visit was the final farewell, before her departure. Peter did not see his mother again until after the war, as a young man in the United States.

During our childhood, Peter rarely shared painful memories. I would hear fleeting mentions at most. But, in our late teens, he apparently believed my brothers and I were ready to hear. On our first trip to Germany, and then more so when I was a college student living in Germany, he talked about his childhood. In the dark corners of a *Ratskeller* (bar), or on the streets of small villages where he grew up, he would tell stories that distracted with humor and legend. He related how as a hungry post-war teen living in a small village he

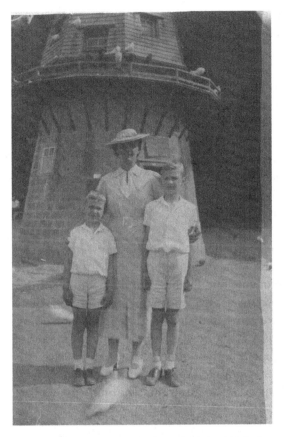

Figure 1.2 Peter (left) and Dieter (right) with their mother Else in Spa, Belgium, shortly before her departure to the United States.

would swim in the local river – the Rhine. He would swim across the river to steal apples from the orchard, then hike back upstream for the return. Or he would hitch rides upriver on barges, from the water. Crazy adventure tales. The hunger – the lack of food – was only given a minor part.

As a teenager, Peter would swim near the Lorelei, a slate outcrop that towers over an S-curve in the Rhine, a site of many boating accidents over the centuries. The translation of Lorelei can be peaceful: a "murmuring rock"; or insidious: a "lurking rock." Folklore has it that a siren, a singing beauty, laid in wait among those rocks and distracted the shipmen. My father relished this tale. The Lorelei tale infiltrated popular culture. Henry Heine wrote a poem about the siren that was included in musical compositions by Shostakovich and others. My father would recite the opening to us, to acquaintances, to dinner guests, first in German then English:

> Ich weiß nicht, was soll es bedeuten,
> Daß ich so traurig bin;
> Ein Märchen aus alten Zeiten,
> Das kommt mir nicht aus dem Sinn.

> I do not know what it means
> That I should feel so sad;
> There is a tale from olden times
> I cannot get out of my mind . . . .

I now realize that, throughout my childhood, my mostly happy father showed glimpses of this melancholy – melancholy tempered with humor and kindness. Did this melancholy motivate him to understand the human brain? He had a lifelong interest in philosophy as well, and in understanding morality and human behavior. Pondering all the children who grow up through a war, as Peter did while witnessing Nazism, it is hard not to think about the impact of these experiences on the development of their brains. We now know from his work that synapses continue to be eliminated throughout childhood, at least through adolescence and likely beyond, refining the neuronal circuits that influence who we are.

References

1. J. Sakai. Core concept: How synaptic pruning shapes neural wiring during development and, possibly, in disease. *Proc Natl Acad Sci USA* 2020; **117**: 16096–9.

2 DISCOVERING SYNAPTIC PRUNING

> For those who think that success in science must be based on aggressive self-promotion and take-no-prisoners competition, Peter Huttenlocher's well-spent life teaches how critical insights can gently but inexorably shift the axis of an entire scientific field, and spill out beyond their own confines to influence society at large.
>
> Chris Walsh, Professor of Pediatrics and Neurology,
> Harvard Medical School, 2013

Peering at thousands of neurons under an electron microscope in the 1970s, Peter sought to understand how the structures through which neurons communicate, known as "synapses," change during development of the human brain. How are these billions of synapses formed and refined? How do these circuits change, and allow us to remember, and to learn? What happens when these connections go awry and what is their relationship to human disease?

The human brain has around 100 billion neurons and each neuron forms multiple branching connections, resulting in roughly a trillion synapses in the adult human brain. In the late 1800s, an improved window into understanding the human brain was enabled by an advance in microscopy and imaging of neurons. The Italian physician Camillo Golgi developed a staining technique using silver nitrate, which enabled a much clearer view of brain cells, known as the "Golgi stain." It densely stains an entire neuron and its long projections, now known as the dendrites and axons. It was a modification of the Golgi stain that Peter and others used 100 years later to uncover new information about how the human brain develops.

Building on Golgi's techniques, in the 1890s Santiago Ramón y Cajal discovered the physical structure of the neuron. A Spanish neuroscientist and artist, Ramón y Cajal is known as the father of modern neuroscience. His groundbreaking studies provided the first window into understanding neuronal connectivity, the basis for human memory. As an artist, Ramón y Cajal drew exquisite and detailed images of everything he saw under the microscope. He defined the neuron as the structural unit of the brain and was the first to visualize the beautiful network of connecting extensions and branches that emanate from the body of a neuron. Some projections, the "axons," tend to be long and relatively unbranched, while others, the "dendrites," are short and highly branched. Ramón y Cajal also described a gap between the axons of one neuron and the dendrites of a neighboring cell as a site of communication between the two cells, later referred to as the synaptic cleft. Axons and dendrites have since been shown to have distinct functions: generally, the dendrites are post-synaptic, or on the receiving end of signals between neurons, and axons are presynaptic, providing the signals that influence the receiving neuron.

In these early years, Ramón y Cajal postulated that the growth of neurons and their ability to form new connections formed the basis for "memory." This was based on the observation that neurons form specific connections with other neurons in a kind of "circuit." He also proposed correctly that information travels in one direction from the axons of one neuron to the dendrites of the neighboring neuron, and that there are specialized functions of neurons. Motor neurons transmit information from the brain to the periphery by, for example, connecting with muscles. Sensory neurons send information from the skin and other peripheral tissue to the brain, to affect brain activity. Other neurons reside in between the motor and sensory neurons and are referred to as "inter-neurons" that provide communication between the sensory and motor neurons. Ramón y Cajal's work and theories are credited with providing the origin for the synaptic theory of memory. Together with Golgi, Ramón y Cajal received the 1906 Nobel Prize in Physiology or Medicine for this groundbreaking work. In 1937, when Peter was just a young boy in Germany, Ramón y Cajal eloquently wrote, "I noticed that every outgrowth, dendritic or axonic, in the course of formation, passes through a chaotic period, so to speak, a period of trials, during which they are sent at random experimental conductors, most of which are destined to disappear." Peter cited this quote in his 2002 book *Neural Plasticity,* as the first reference to the idea of synaptic elimination [1].

The gaps between the axons and dendrites of neurons were referred to as a "synapse" by the English physiologist Charles Sherrington. Sherrington received the Nobel Prize in Physiology or Medicine in 1932 for showing that reflexes (think of the human knee reflex) are not a simple arc of connectivity but rather derive from integrated networks of activation between neurons. He demonstrated that some neurons excite other neurons, while others inhibit the activity of neurons, thereby enabling a coordinated and integrated response. As part of this work, Sherrington proposed the idea of "synaptic communication" between neurons.

The idea that neurons communicate, and regulate the activity of other neurons, paved the way for the evolving concept that these connections can change over time based on their input and experience. Neural plasticity or brain plasticity is defined as the ability of the nervous system to adapt by reorganizing its structure, connectivity and function in response to both external and internal stimuli. This concept of plasticity was raised in the fields of both psychology and neuroscience as early as the 1890s. Credit for the specific term "neural plasticity" has been given to the Polish neuroscientist Jerzy Konorski.

When Peter launched his work on synapses in the developing human brain, it was not known how these connections change during human development. However, the idea that synaptic changes underlie brain plasticity was gaining traction during the 1960s and 1970s. The work of David Hubel and Torsten Wiesel elegantly displayed the plasticity of the developing non-adult brain. Using sensory deprivation in kittens, Hubel and Wiesel deprived one eye of visual input from birth by sewing it closed and then recorded the activity of neurons on both sides of the brain. To the surprise of Hubel, Wiesel and their colleagues worldwide, a few months after blocking input to one eye, all neurons on both sides of the "striate cortex" responded to input from the intact eye [2]. It was expected that the part of the brain that would have responded to the closed eye would have remained quiescent. But instead, some brain areas previously quiescent due to sensory deprivation had regained activity when studied months after the start of the deprivation. The open eye had co-opted some of the synaptic inputs from the closed eye, on the opposite side of the brain, as part of a rewiring of synaptic connectivity. This provided direct evidence that the visual cortical area of the brain is rewired due to the visual deprivation in one eye. It also raised critical questions about how environmental changes lead to a competition between synaptic connections and their remodeling.

The work of Hubel and Wiesel revealed that the plasticity and reorganization of the visual cortex only occurred during a limited developmental window of the kitten, referred to as the "critical period." If the same experiment was done in older cats, the sensory deprivation did not lead to a change in cortical connectivity and rewiring [3]. Hubel and Wiesel also performed reverse suturing by opening the previously deprived eye and covering the dominant eye. As long as this was done in the first months of life, during this critical period the newly uncovered eye co-opted the wiring of the ocular dominance pattern, switching the "visual activity" to the uncovered eye that was now receiving the input. These findings suggested that there was something unique about younger animals which allowed for rewiring of neuronal connectivity leading to functional plasticity.

It was precisely these questions about neuronal connectivity that Peter aimed to understand in the early 1970s. In addition to his scientific work,

Peter was busy running an active pediatric neurology practice and making substantial medical school teaching and medical resident training contributions at Yale University and then the University of Chicago. It was logical to be drawn primarily to studying brain tissues from human patients with pathologies. Through his work in the first half of the 1970s, Peter discovered that there was stunted development and abnormal shape of synapses from children with significant developmental delay [4]. This dendritic spine "dysgenesis" provided support for the idea that the shape of synapses, and not just the number of synapses, is a factor to consider when studying the plasticity of the human brain.

Using specimens obtained from autopsies, Peter studied the brains of children who had intellectual disabilities, comparing them to samples from children with "normal" development who had died for other reasons. He undertook a painstaking set of studies using an electron microscope to acquire hundreds of images from specific brain regions. He then scrutinized photographic prints of the electron microscope images and counted neurons and synaptic junctions by hand (Figure 2.1). Peter found something interesting in the "normal" brain samples. He realized that to understand what went awry with disease he first had to understand what happened during normal human brain development. Peter later said that "the findings in the normal population were more interesting than the abnormal population." By the 1970s,

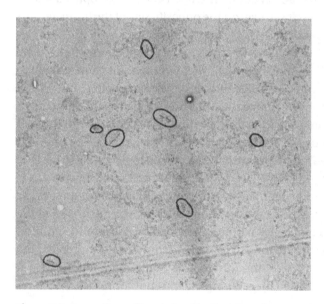

Figure 2.1 Synaptic profiles stained by the phosphotungstic acid method (PTA). Image is from Peter Huttenlocher's personal collection of the images of synapses used for quantification. Seven identifiable synapses were circled on the image.

when Peter was doing this work, much of the work emanating from molecular bioscience laboratories was being done by graduate students, postdoctoral trainees and scientific staff, working under the direction of a lead scientist. Hearkening back to the days of Golgi and Ramón y Cajal, Peter instead did much of this seminal work himself. One of Peter's former trainees, Dr. Carter Snead (Professor of Pediatrics, Neurology and Pharmacology, University of Toronto), commented that Peter "did it the hard way." He spent hours at the microscope, analyzing brain samples. It was daunting to collect the samples, and to perform the analysis of synapse numbers in a tiny region of the brain. What did it mean to look at such a small piece of tissue when the human brain was much larger? Could you accurately quantify synapses in these samples? There were many hurdles and more questions than answers as Peter embarked upon this work.

In his landmark single-authored paper published in *Brain Research* in 1979 [5], Peter reported on changes in synaptic density in a region of the human cerebral cortex in individuals with no intellectual disabilities. He had found something entirely unexpected. Early results had led him to broaden the study; autopsy specimens were now used from the newborn period to advanced adulthood. He observed that synaptic density in the adults was relatively constant, with some decline at older ages (74–90). At the time of birth, the number of synapses was already high in infants, comparable to the adults, although the morphology of the synapses was different in infants than in adults, suggesting functional differences. During the first months of life, there is robust production of new synapses – to levels 50% greater than the adult brain. The number of synapses peaks during childhood and then regresses. What was most surprising was the elimination of many of these synapses during the subsequent childhood years, a prolonged period of intense learning, up until late adolescence or even adulthood (Figure 2.2). Peter wrote that "the human cerebral cortex is one of a number of neuronal systems in which loss of neurons and synapses appears to occur as a late developmental event." He showed for the first time that there is elimination or "pruning" of synapses that coincides with key developmental milestones in childhood such as learning to walk or speak. The overall number of synaptic connections goes down, not up, as we learn and remember. Synaptic connections are not just refined. As part of healthy brain development, millions of synapses are pruned away and lost.

Since the time of Peter's discovery of synaptic pruning in childhood, and the work of Hubel and Wiesel, there has been substantial progress in understanding how neuronal activity influences synaptic pruning in mammals. This activity-dependent synaptic pruning occurs in the developing nervous system through the effects of both spontaneous neuronal activity and activity induced

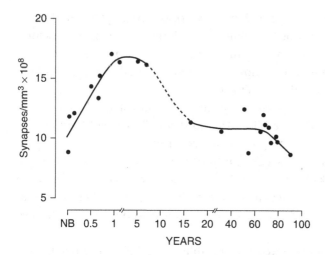

Figure 2.2 Synapse counts from the middle frontal gyrus, showing reduction of synapses with age – the figure that is most frequently shown by other scientists. From: Huttenlocher PR. 1979. Synaptic density in human frontal cortex – developmental changes and effects of aging. *Brain Res* 163:195–205. doi: 10.1016/0006-8993(79)90349-4. Reprinted with permission.

by sensory experiences, such as visual or auditory input. Synapses that are stimulated and active are maintained while the quiescent synapses are eliminated during this developmental rewiring of neuronal circuits in the brain. As an example, in work done in the 1980s by Shatz and colleagues, the impact of neural activity on synaptic elimination during development was directly demonstrated [6]. The retinal cells in the eye extend axons to a structure in the brain known as the lateral geniculate nucleus (LGN). In the LGN, the retinal axons branch and form exuberant synapses during development. Subsequently, these robust branches and synapses in the LGN are pruned and refined to form an organized visual map. The neurons that respond to a particular stimulus are co-localized in specific areas of the LGN. But when neural activity is blocked synaptic pruning fails, leading to a disorganized network of branching axons and synapses in the LGN and, as a result, a tangled visual map. In recent decades, our understanding of the molecular underpinnings of activity-dependent synaptic pruning has exploded and this work has uncovered an elegant multi-tiered system that regulates synaptic pruning during development.

However, at the time of Peter's discovery of synaptic pruning, widespread recognition by neuroscientists did not quickly follow. While the discoveries fascinated Peter and a cohort of scientists, their reports on the work, like the work of Hubel and Wiesel, were submitted for publication to respected but less widely read specialist journals. Peter gave a number of invited talks internationally about his findings – again, usually to specialist audiences. There were some arranged media interviews orchestrated by the University of Chicago, which were picked up by German newspapers including *Die Welt* – a pleasing bit of recognition. One of Peter's sons, who was visiting family in Munich in the summer of 1978, wrote, "Dad: you were on page one of *Die Welt* in Deutschland, re: work on brain development. Oma H [Peter's stepmother] suggested maybe you would win a Nobel prize – they were impressed." However, it took many years and much creative work for an increasing number of neuroscience and psychology experts to absorb, validate, rediscover, expand upon and more widely publicize the core ideas of synaptic pruning.

As neuroscientist Christian Hansel (2021) noted in his book entitled *Memory Makes the Brain: The Biological Machinery That Uses Experiences to Shape Individual Brains* [7]:

[Hubel and Wiesel] performed much of their work alone . . . and published their most important work in a few papers that were published . . . in journals that focused on science as opposed to flashy headlines . . . . This was true of Peter Huttenlocher as well. Yet, all three of them were giants in their fields and left a mark on neuroscience like few others.

In an obituary for Peter Huttenlocher published in *Nature* in 2013 [8], Professor Chris Walsh of Harvard University said:

Huttenlocher's discovery that synapses are overproduced and then pruned was 20 years or more ahead of its time. Today, most ideas about human brain development, from the microscopic to the macroscopic to the societal, draw on his work. For instance, researchers are now investigating the mechanisms that control pruning, the possibilities that this synaptic plasticity provides, and how to use an understanding of synaptic development to optimize early educational intervention, language learning or music instruction.

Dr. Jeffrey Lichtman, a developmental neurobiologist at Harvard who uses sophisticated computer imagery to map brain circuitry, said to the *New York Times* (August 26, 2013):

Here's a person who was looking for the physical underpinnings of abnormalities of brain function, and that is a difficult thing to do even today . . . . It's still a central challenge in brain science and here was a person who was years ahead, decades ahead of his time.

References

1. P. R. Huttenlocher. *Neural Plasticity: The Effects of Environment on the Development of the Cerebral Cortex.* Harvard University Press, 2002.
2. T. N. Wiesel and D. H. Hubel. Effects of visual deprivation on morphology and physiology of cells in the cats lateral geniculate body. *J Neurophysiol* 1963; **26**: 978–93.
3. D. H Hubel and T. N. Wiesel. The period of susceptibility to the physiological effects of unilateral eye closure in kittens. *J Physiol* 1970; **206(2)**: 419–36.
4. P. R. Huttenlocher. Synaptic and dendritic development and mental defect. *UCLA Forum Med Sci* 1975; **18**: 123–40.
5. P. R. Huttenlocher, Synaptic density in human frontal cortex: Developmental changes and effects of aging. *Brain Res* 1979; **163**: 195–205.
6. D. Sretavan and C. J. Shatz, Prenatal development of individual retinogeniculate axons during the period of segregation. *Nature* 1984; **308**: 845–8.
7. C. Hansel. *Memory Makes the Brain: The Biological Machinery That Uses Experiences to Shape Individual Brains.* World Scientific, 2021.
8. C. A. Walsh. Peter Huttenlocher (1931–2013). *Nature* 2013; **502**: 7470.

3 ELSE, PETER'S MOTHER

I was put in this world to change it
                Kathe Kollwitz, German artist (1867–1945)

Any understanding of Peter, and his motivation to figure out how the human brain develops and can go awry in disease, requires delving into his childhood and the lives of his parents. Peter was particularly inspired by his mother, who was guided by the "need to be good" and spoke out against Nazism while most people remained silent. Peter's mother, Else Lamparter, was born in 1904 in Ohringen, a medieval village in the rolling hills of southwest Germany. As an only child, she was doted on by her parents and her "Uncle" Uhle. Her family ran an expediting business transporting luggage and goods from the local rail station. As a child, Peter visited his grandparents in the summers and helped his soft-spoken grandfather with the horses and carts as they traveled through the hilly cobbled streets of Ohringen. The Lamparter family had large, lively social gatherings with family and friends, which were documented in the many family photographs.

The family lived in a house on the top of a hill in Ohringen. Else's mom, Peter's Oma, was stern and commanded respect while Uncle Uhle provided a balance of humor and wit. These contrasts were apparent in the pair of painted portraits that sparked conversation and intrigue for decades after. In Oma Lamparter's portrait she looks directly at people, commanding notice from the living room wall. Austere, she sits erect against a red velvet backdrop, holding a pink flower bouquet in her arms. Her strong blue eyes meet those of every viewer from all perspectives in the room. On another wall hangs Uncle Uhle, posed with a friendly smile and holding a pipe, his eyes gazing into the distance. Uncle Uhle – not literally an uncle – was a source of curiosity for friends and family. When asked about Uncle Uhle, Peter would simply answer, with a glint in his eye, "Uncle Uhle lived with my grandparents." When the curious pushed further, one never got a clear answer, just a quiet, quizzical smile.

Else grew into an adult during the Weimar period in Germany. After the First World War, the Treaty of Versailles imposed harsh restrictions on Germany as its government transitioned from a monarchy to a republic. The Weimar Republic, Germany's first democracy, was formed in 1918. This parliamentary government was handicapped from the beginning during a time of economic turmoil and unrest. It was also a time of social change in Germany: for the first time, women had the right to vote and hold office. There was "free speech," with newspapers publishing the views of social democrats, Nazis and communists. The political climate gave rise to an astounding number of political parties and viewpoints, unable to achieve any form of consensus.

During this tumultuous but relatively progressive time, the arts, sciences and music flourished. The government allowed Jewish scientists, such as Albert Einstein, to hold positions at German universities for the first time. By the early 1920s, the Weimar Republic stabilized, and Germany experienced improved economic conditions and improved foreign relations. It was a time of new ideas and intellectual freedom for artists, scientists and musicians. Famous artistic initiatives included the Bauhaus arts and crafts school in Berlin and the studio of the film company UFA New Objectivity artists (Neue Sachlickeit). Expressionist art also thrived during the Weimar period. Egon Schiele, Wassilly Kandinsky, Max Beckman and others generated angst-filled art that reflected the turmoil of the time. Kathe Kollwitz translated this into works of social protest including poignant and dark images of starving children and prisoners of war. Notwithstanding the free society that enabled the rise of expressionism, many Germans viewed the artistic movement and other Weimar - period ideas as immoral and decadent.

During this period of artistic innovation and experimentation in Germany, Else developed into a talented performer. From Ohringen, she then studied at the Stuttgart Conservatory. Richard Huttenlocher, an engineering and chemistry student, fell in love with Else (Figure 3.1). After a fast romance they were married in 1925 in Stuttgart. A family portrait of Else shows a beautiful young woman with red lipstick coyly displaying an engagement ring, as she gazes into the distance. Decades later, family members still recalled how heads would turn when Else entered a room.

Women gained more power in the Weimar republic: not only the right to vote but also the right to work. Outspoken self-determination was not uncommon. It was in this environment that Else grew up, attended university and continued to work after marrying and having children. But it was a minority of women in Germany who accepted this newfound freedom and many men also resented this "progress." Economic uncertainty grew in Germany and abroad in the late 1920s, and discomfort with the "new woman" was one of many factors that contributed to the fall of the Weimar Republic and the rise of Nazism. Dieter was born in 1928 and Peter in 1931. Throughout this time, Else starred as a dramatic soprano in the Cologne opera. Richard worked as

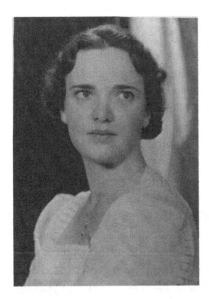

Figure 3.1 Peter's mother Else, around the time of her marriage to Richard in the late 1920s.

a chemist at a chemical company nearby and they lived in a town along the Rhine, Oberlahnstein. With two successful careers and two young children, Else and Richard exemplified a "modern German" family.

Else and Richard also maintained a dynamic group of musician and scientist friends, many of whom were Jewish. The owners of Richard's chemical company were Jewish. William Steinberg, a world-famous Jewish conductor, was Else's mentor at the Cologne Conservatory. He also offered Else a position singing in the Frankfort opera, where he was lead conductor. But then in 1933, the opera relieved Steinberg of his position in Frankfort because he was Jewish. Outraged, Else protested Steinberg's dismissal, something that Peter often spoke proudly of. Else refused to join the music guild and Nazi party. For a Wagnerian opera singer, a lead performer of music that was revered by Hitler, she staked out a particularly dangerous position.

By the mid-1930s, much life in Germany was dominated by fear. Nazi informants were everywhere. The culture of intimidation was pervasive. Whether in cities or smaller towns, people had reason to be terrified. The mayor of a town next to Oberlahnstein was publicly executed by hanging in the town center in 1936 because he supported the local Jewish families and was deemed to be deviant and not "loyal" to Nazism.

Else and Richard responded to the fear differently. Else stubbornly spoke out. Richard hated Nazism and never joined the party, but he was quiet. The son of a former policeman, Richard was careful. This – surely among other things –

led to significant tension in their relationship. Many years later, in a letter
dated September 1, 1949, Richard wrote to Else and spoke of their relationship:

> I tried hard to find the way for both boys to prepare them for a good life together
> with you – so they never heard a bad word about you from me. They know that we
> lived our own lives and because of that we parted from one another. I also tried to
> make it clear that one has to respect the life of every person. And also awoke their
> understanding that it is better to separate from a marriage than try and live a life
> together where you would just squash each other.

Richard had relationships outside of the marriage. In the divorce decree it
stated, "Since the end of July 1935 the 'plaintiff' Richard does not contest the anti-
matrimonial relations with Trude Miller, that they continued after the last marital
act." The document noted that both Else and Richard had "social contacts with
Jewish people, as for instance, the owner of the chemical company, where the
plaintiff was employed as Chief chemist . . . Dr. Beckenheimer, a Jewish physician,
had come to the home frequently in the capacity of doctor to the older son." Both
Else and Richard shared responsibility for the disintegration of their relationship.

Before the divorce agreement was finalized, Richard and Else both felt
increasingly insecure in their small village along the Rhine. Richard moved
with his young sons to the eastern region of Germany, to the town of Greiz,
which had a different branch of the same chemical company. In part, this
allowed him to escape the skeptical views of their neighbors in Oberlahnstein.
Else fled to Belgium and then France. She never returned to Germany.

A letter from Dieter and Peter to their mother and grandmother marks their
new life in Greiz with their father and new "mom." Around the same time, Else
departed France to travel to the United States.

Greiz, December 29, 1937

Dear Mom and Grandma!

Thank you very much for the stationery, the book, the bicycle lamp, the
stamps, the little bags, the sweater, and the pants, which are much too big
for me. We had our own little Christmas tree where we gave presents to dad
and mom. Peter thanks you for the stationery, the two books, the little bags,
the sweater, the stamps and the jacket. How are you? We are fine. We have
a big board now and it sits on the table and on it we built the [wooden toy]
train and we don't need to slide on the floor anymore.

Many greetings and kisses

And a happy new year,

Dieter and Peter

Else Lamparter in the United States

Designated as a "German refugee," Else traveled by US luxury liner, the SS *Washington*, from France to the United States in January 1938. She departed from LeHavre, France, and traveled alone. An anonymous wealthy American family, who supported the transit of German refugees, funded her transport. The luxury of her travel was documented in the elaborate menus, describing the evening multi-course meals, that she saved from her transit. The donors also supported the transit of her piano to the United States, the treasured musical instrument from her childhood. Else Huttenlocher arrived in New York City through Ellis Island on January 6, 1938.

Else then changed her name to Else Lamparter, her maiden name, and lived for the first year in New York City. She cleaned homes for wealthy New York families. Soon after arriving in the United States, she sang for her host family. They were delighted and connected her with the NBC program *Major Bowes Amateur Hour* – a type of *American Idol* talent search of the 1930s and 1940s. Frank Sinatra was discovered on this show.

A handwritten letter written shortly after Else's arrival praised her performance on the show:

Thursday evening June 22, 1938

NBC network Major Bowes Radio
To Miss Else Lamparter
My dear madam
   I heard you sing last night and it was divinely beautiful. You have an exquisite lyric quality that lingers in the memory long after the song is finished.
   Why I should write you about my enjoyment I do not quite know. Being of the vast silent audience that seldom indulges in personal comment.
However, I sense that I should pay you this courtesy of sincere appreciation. You deserve it. And perhaps you have won it by your courageous attitude.

Else "won" the competition. The performances on *Major Bowes Amateur Hour* connected Else again with her friend and former conductor in Cologne William Steinberg, who was conducting the New York NBC Symphony. Steinberg subsequently became a frequent guest conductor for the New York Philharmonic and a friend of Leonard Bernstein. As the war progressed and in the early postwar years, both Steinberg and Bernstein made entreaties to promote Else's singing career in New York City. However, Else had other ideas. She decided that the demanding life of an opera singer would not allow her to reunite with her children. She needed a financially stable home and life in the United States. To achieve this, she moved to a smaller town in western New York State to teach voice lessons. In the 1940 US census, Else Lamparter, aged 35, was listed as a "lodger" with the Schultz family in Erie, NY. Her vocation was singer and vocal instructor.

In the United States, Else continued her criticism of Nazism and described the conditions for families in Germany. In November 1939, the *Dunkirk Evening Observer* reported her speaking event at the Adams Memorial Church, about education in Germany under:

> *Miss Lamparter, recently arrived in this country from Europe, told of Germany's system and operation of schools. The attendance was large, numbering 90 parents and friends. Miss Else Lamparter of Gowanda – recently of Germany, gave an interesting and informal presentation based on personal knowledge, to illustrate this point: A child was punished at home, by his parents, for a misbehavior. The child complained to Nazi leaders of the act, and the parents were sent to a concentration camp as punishment for interfering with the state.*

Else later wrote an updated, more complete, telling, which was found in her personal collection, entitled "Education in Germany":

> *Several years ago, I was asked to give a lecture on "Education in Germany" and I felt quite embarrassed about it because I had never made a speech before. Generally, girls in Germany stay in the background and leave the "big word" to the men-folks, but I accepted nonetheless, because the offer thrilled me.*
>
> *If I want to give you a picture about education in Germany I can't help but speak about the difference in education before the Third Reich and under the ideas of Nazism. It is not so much a change in the method of teaching as in the matter of thought and customs of living.*
>
> *The children of my generation were not brought up with politics. They were unburdened with the exception of the world war – not thinking about race differences and not taught that Germany is the greatest country in the world, surrounded by nations which want to destroy her on account of fear of her strength and her population's intelligence. So, we did not have planted into our minds the feeling of over-estimation and the need to self-defend in the same breath. We – first – were children, our parent's children, looking up to them, and then second, we were Germans. Germany's youth today belong to the state and the parents do not have the right and the courage any more to influence their children's way of education, line of thought and behavior. For it happened that children punished by their parents on account of bad behavior, reported them to*

their group leaders, who are selected Nazis, and the result was that their father or mother took a trip to the Concentration Camp. The children are not to blame for that. They have the task to look out for the Nazi-enemies and many of them do not even stop for their parents or relatives, because the reward for getting good points is too tempting.

That part of children's time which is not occupied by school work has to be devoted to the Nazi party, instead of spending the leisure hours in the family or in the youth movements of girl or boy scouts, Wandervögel ["wandering birds"] or the various youth groups sponsored by the churches, as Germany had before Hitlerism. The privacy is taken away by uniforms for girls and boys. Today it is obligatory that each pure-Aryan child has to join the Jungvokl [young people] or the Bund Deutscher Mädchen [Bund of German girls] at the age of 10; at the age of 14 boys join the Hitler-Jugend [Hitler Youth]. The aim of these youth organizations is to enlist and train youth for the impersonal attachment of the state and their detachment from the personal family home. Already at the tender age of 6 or sooner the educators try to teach the children idolizing the Führer [leader]. As soon as they have to join the youth organizations, at age 10, the active work for the party starts. From then on the children are under the constant supervision of the party. They have to attend political meetings, they have to listen in closed formation to every speech of the leading men – personally if possible or over the radio – they have to do street service on collection days. They have club meetings in the evening and listen to propaganda speeches of visiting potentates. The weekend is devoted to military drill through every detail of military life. Every boy must be able to march with a 11 pound pack from 10 to 13 miles a day. Neither rain shower nor sunshine will free them – according to the Spartan Law – only the strong ones have a right to survive – the weak ones may perish.

We cannot know the extent to which thoughts of her sons affected her expressions about the situation in Germany, but the scenario of youth indoctrination and cultivation as informants was unfortunately common in Germany at the time. Although now in the United States, Else knew what it was like to have lived in fear, and to have her family, passport and safety taken away by Nazism. What she did not know at the time was that Richard took the risk of speaking openly against Nazism to his children.

One of the few things Else brought with her with from Europe, in addition to her piano, was her original copy of *Der Hirt auf dem Felsen* (The Shepherd on the Rock), a multi-section lied or song for soprano by Franz Schubert. She would play and sing this lied throughout her life.

The following are two sections for the song:

Karl August Varnhagen – "Nächtlicher Schall" (Nocturnal sound)

> In tiefem Gram verzehr ich mich,
> Mir ist die Freude hin,
> Auf Erden mir die Hoffnung wich,
> Ich hier so einsam bin.
>
> I am consumed in misery,
> Happiness is far from me,
> Hope has on earth eluded me,
> I am so lonesome here.
>
> So sehnend klang im Wald das Lied,
> So sehnend klang es durch die Nacht,
> Die Herzen es zum Himmel zieht
> Mit wunderbarer Macht.
>
> So longingly did sound the song,
> So longingly through wood and night,
> Towards heaven it draws all hearts
> With amazing strength.

Wilhelm Müller – "Liebesgedanken" (Thoughts of love)

> Der Frühling will kommen,
> Der Frühling, meine Freud',
> Nun mach' ich mich fertig
> Zum Wandern bereit
>
> The Springtime will come,
> The Springtime, my happiness,
> Now must I make ready
> To wander forth.

All was not well with Else in her early years in the United States. She was not happy being separated from her children, and she was worried that her children would forget her. She also feared for her children and their indoctrination into Nazism. In February 1940, she wrote in a letter to her mother:

As you can imagine I am very upset by the whole situation and depressed that I cannot even take pleasure in the music. And, on those days that I am totally incapable to even sing – it is a dreadful thought to know you are all surrounded by these worries. I do not know what is happening to my children and that makes my heart heavier and heavier. And so, I am afraid this letter will not bring much sunshine into your house – not because I am not well but because what is happening in the old world – and who is looking after my nearest loved ones – it has taken all of my joy. From the kids, I have not heard since my birthday letter which arrived much later – no Christmas greeting. Of course, I am clever enough to assume it is due to the difficult mail passage and situations – rather to blame them for not writing. I presume Richard has his hands and head full with other things at the moment. It will be important for you to talk to them about me so that they will not forget their mother – that she loves them dearly and she thinks about them every day. They accompany me into my sleep and dreams ....

She wrote a poem in English during this time:

> None but humans
> Feel sorrow and joy,
> Are elated by beauty,
> Emotion supreme.
> Chosen are those
> Endowed to perceive
> A small bloom's perfection,
> The obvious in arts.

In spite of this Else did wander forth, and she continued to perform, as reported in the *Buffalo Courier Express* on Monday January 9, 1939:

Operatic soprano presents program: more than 200 at event

Miss Else Lamparter of New York City formerly dramatic soprano of the Cologne Opera Company of Germany.

The Delaware avenue clubhouse was decorated most attractively with vases of fresh flowers placed at vantage points throughout the lower floors. Miss Lamparter's presentation of Dichtheure Halle from Wagner's opera Tannhauser and the aria Pamina from Mozart's magic flute were received with enthusiasm. The attractive singer was wearing a molded gown of black satin, with a square neckline and flowing hemline.

It was during one of these performances that she met Max, a fellow 1930s German immigrant, a Buffalo NY pediatrician and her future husband. Max was of Jewish descent but not from a religious family. Max had a daughter Eva from his first marriage, born in Germany in 1926. Eva's mother was also Jewish, but she had passed away when Eva was young and Max had remarried in Germany to a non-Jewish woman. By all reports she was a nice stepmother to Eva. Max always claimed that he did not feel particularly threatened while in Germany – perhaps because he was married to a non-Jewish woman, and also because of his status as a practicing physician. But by 1936 his nephews in the United States read the situation differently and, after multiple efforts, convinced Max that he had to leave. Max's second marriage dissolved. The nephews arranged and sponsored the passage of Max and Eva to the United States by boat.

Else Lamparter became a naturalized citizen of the United States in 1943. On her citizenship application she listed her "minor" children Peter and Dieter. Citizenship was automatic for the minor children of American citizens (less than 21 at the time). She was now determined to work toward the transit of her children to the United States, before they turned 21. She needed a stable family environment to petition for her sons to join her in the United States. Conveniently, and genuinely (one can say based on their subsequent 25 years together), she had formed a loving relationship with Max Landsburger.

In the late summer of 1943, Max's daughter Eva, an accomplished violinist, headed off to college at the Oberlin Conservatory of Music. A few months later, the local paper announced that:

> *Miss Else Lamparter, of Silver Creek, choir director for the past year of the First Methodist church of Dunkirk, will be married in Buffalo, Saturday, October 28, to Dr. Max Landsberger, associate assistant of pediatrics at the Deaconess hospital and physician at the division of child's hygiene department of health, Buffalo. Miss Lamparter is one of the outstanding vocalists and teachers in this vicinity.*

After marriage, Else's family in Germany remained a primary focus. Multiple letters and documents show her ongoing efforts to get Peter and Dieter to the United States. But, in the mid-1940s, Peter and Dieter were children in the midst of a war. Travel was not possible.

Else continued to sing in Buffalo. A notice from the Buffalo Museum of Science in 1943 now listed her singing as Else Landsburger. William Steinberg, Else's mentor and conductor from Cologne, moved to Buffalo and served as music director of the Buffalo Philharmonic Orchestra from 1945 until 1952. Else remained lifelong friends with Steinberg, and Max and Else frequently socialized with Steinberg and his wife. They also befriended the composer Paul Hindemith, who taught at the University of Buffalo in the 1940s before moving to Yale. Paul Hindemith had also fled Germany, because the government discredited his "modern" music, which it viewed as a threat to Nazism.

Else performed on several occasions with the Buffalo Philharmonic when Steinberg was lead conductor. After Buffalo, Steinberg spent many years as the music director of the Pittsburgh Symphony and conducted extended engagements with both the London Philharmonic and the Boston Symphony Orchestra.

Her last documented official performance occasioned this announcement:

Buffalo philharmonic orchestra 4th symphony concert
  William Steinberg music director 1947
  Else Landsburger, soloist.

More than 10 years after Else departed LeHavre for the United States, Peter and Dieter traveled from Germany to reunite with their mother. Peter could now communicate with his mother in person rather than through constrained letter-writing, and hear his mother's tales. They moved in with Else and Max at the end of December 1948, shortly before Peter's 18th birthday.

4 RICHARD, PETER'S FATHER, AND PETER'S UNCLE FRITZ

The world will not be destroyed by those who do evil, but by those who watch them without doing anything.

Albert Einstein, theoretical physicist (1879–1955)

Peter's father, Richard Huttenlocher, was born in 1900 in Alte Weinsteige, in the hilly vineyards near Stuttgart. Richard's father, Johann Huttenlocher, was a policeman in Stuttgart. Richard's mother, Elisabethe, "Oma" Huttenlocher (family name Gaupp), was a doting mother and ran a traditional home, with a knack for German baking that she shared with her grandson Peter. Both Richard and his older brother Friedrich (Uncle Fritz) studied the sciences in the *Gymnasium* (high school), but their studies were interrupted by the First World War. Fritz was stationed at the western front from 1914 to 1918, where he was wounded, and was recognized with an Iron Cross from the Prussian government. Richard had only a brief stint as a young soldier, toward the end of the war. After the war, they both returned to live at the family home. Richard studied chemistry at the University of Stuttgart and Fritz studied geography/geology at the University of Tübingen. They both married young. Fritz married his wife Hannah, a traditional woman, in 1920, and continued to work at the University of Tübingen as a lecturer and then professor.

Richard, the second son, was more independent - minded and embraced the freedoms of Weimar Germany. He fell in love with Else, the rebellious and strong-minded young opera student. They were quickly married and shortly after welcomed their first son Dieter. After completing his PhD, Richard left the family home and moved to Oberlahnstein for his work at a chemical company while Else sang with the Cologne Opera. Shortly after their departure in 1931, around the time of Peter's birth, Richard's father passed away. As a child, Peter frequently visited his Oma and Uncle Fritz and their large dogs. From their home you could walk for miles on trails through the vineyards, with expansive views of the valley below. There were frequent family visits to the large extended Huttenlocher and Gaupp families, who lived near Stuttgart, in the village of Beutelsbach. Indeed, the Huttenlocher family can be traced to a small village in the region starting in the mid-1400s.

Uncle Fritz was an artist and an outdoors enthusiast who enjoyed hiking with his young nephews in the German Alps. Peter recalled hikes with his uncle as a child, an interest that he shared with his own children years later in the United States. There are scant details of how Peter's extended family lived during the war. Fritz was a teacher and professor at the University of Tübingen and a leader in dissecting the geography and geological features of the Bavarian Alps. An online resource from the "Commission for the Geographic History of Baden-Wurttemberg" provides some information about his success as a geographer "as well as his highly artistic disposition, to which his numerous paintings, especially his landscape paintings, testify in their immediate and sure grasp of form and color. Initially, he even wavered as to whether he should follow the path of an artist or that of a scientist." Fritz Huttenlocher took on the major part of southwestern Germany in the great joint work that German geographers undertook immediately after the Second World War. He was interested in cultural landscapes and how populations settled and formed towns in these geographical regions. It was also noted that "through the solid training of student teachers, who revered him as a competent, open-minded, always helpful, kind academic teacher, he had an extraordinarily broad impact."

Fritz's involvement with the Nazis generated some family disagreement. How Fritz responded to Richard and to Else, who openly opposed Nazism in the early 1930s, remains unclear. However, the brothers remained close with frequent family visits (Figure 4.1). But as time passed, Richard avoided the Nazi party with dogged determination. Peter struggled to reconcile his fondness for his "kind" Uncle Fritz with his uncle's activities during the war. It was compulsory under Nazism that all professors join and serve the party to continue employment at the university. In the same source, it is documented that Friedrich Huttenlocher served from "1939–1945 Military service, and from 1941 as a military geographer; Captain of the reserves." As in so many German families, this was not spoken of. After the war, Uncle Fritz and many other academics in Germany continued in their academic positions as if Nazism had not happened. The war years were shrouded in a zone of silence.

Richard worked in the private sector and party membership was not required. As Peter's half-brother Wolfgang later described, even when Nazi officials appeared at his home to encourage party membership, he declined to join. Richard was remembered as a person who was always thinking ahead, considering all options and planning. As a chemist, he was expected to aid in the war effort through the production of ammunitions in their company

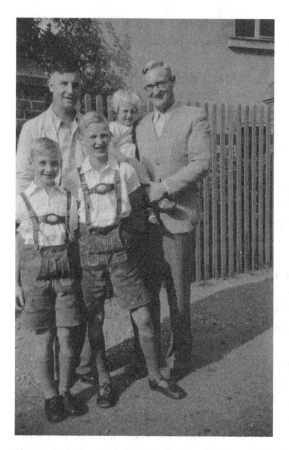

Figure 4.1 Peter's Uncle Fritz (left) and father Richard holding his younger brother Wolfgang. Peter (left) and Dieter (right).

factories that normally produced soaps and surfactants. He did the work, but he would not go as far as taking an oath of loyalty to Hitler. And although it was dangerous to do so, he communicated his disdain to his sons. As he wrote to Else after the war when helping to prepare her for Dieter and Peter's arrival in her home: "You must keep in front of your eyes that both boys were raised in a constant dismissal and critique of Nazism – both were brought up to deny and criticize the national socialism. They were brought up to disagree with the government."

Richard also wrote the following to Else in 1949, after Peter and his brother had emigrated, perhaps as part of a coming to terms with his own actions over the previous 15 years: "In the German concentration camps many found their end in a most terrible way. All of us really did not know whether we would not have to share the same end. When we disagreed then hell broke loose." Else had been labeled deviant. She had openly defied and protested Nazism. Many "deviant" citizens were imprisoned and murdered. There was a fine line between deviant defiance and inconspicuous defiance. Quiet refusal to join the party was generally not met with imprisonment, at least for less prominent citizens. Richard had remained in Germany while Else fled, placing an ocean between herself and Germany but also her two children. Richard, we will see, schemed a bit. He survived and raised a family. He rejected Nazism in private but, as a chemist, also did his national duty for the war effort.

5 GREIZ: KRIEGSKINDER (CHILDREN OF WAR)

Greiz is a town along the White Eister River on the eastern edge of Thuringia, a few kilometers from Saxony and 50 kilometers from the Czech Republic. The town square is next to an expansive English garden, with a castle looming on the hill above. This region of Thuringia is known for its many forests and mountains. It is also known for its ancient cities and the Wartburg Castle, which is now a UNESCO World Heritage Site.

In 1936, Richard arranged a work transfer from his chemical company in Lahnstein to the branch of Zschimmer and Schwarz in the Greiz area. He was in his mid-30s, divorced, with the custody of two young sons, fleeing his home. It was too uncomfortable, and possibly dangerous, for Richard to remain in Oberlahnstein. As stated in the divorce decree, Richard had "social contacts with Jewish people." Else was a Jewish sympathizer and had fled to Belgium. In Greiz, 400 km away, no one knew Richard or Else. It was a fresh start. Richard's cousin, called Tante Minna by the boys, moved with Richard and the boys to Greiz. Minna had lost her husband in the First World War and, as a widow, was eager to help Richard with the boys. Tante Minna was loving and provided needed care in the absence of Dieter and Peter's mother.

Shortly after arriving in Greiz, Richard met Charlotte Limmer, the 19-year-old daughter of a fabric maker in Greiz. Once again, the romance was fast and they were married in 1937. Peter's brother Wolfgang arrived in 1937 and Götz in 1940. Germany, having taken over Czechoslovakia, invaded Poland in the interim. Charlotte became the young mother of four boys in the midst of a war that was increasing in scale. Germany conducted blitzkrieg invasions of Belgium and France in 1940, and France surrendered just six weeks later. The bombing of London occurred in the fall of 1940. Wolfgang described Richard as a "family man" who tried to make things as "normal" as possible for the children. Richard arranged summer trips for the family in Zingst, on the sea, with Tante Minna. Photographs show the four boys, with Charlotte, playing on the beach in 1941 (Figure 5.1). Peter was 10 years old. This was the last time the

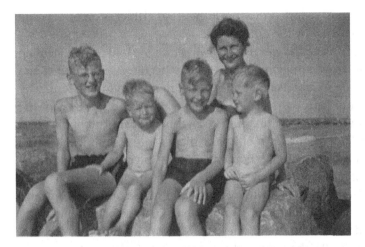

Figure 5.1 Peter, his stepmother and the boys. From left, Dieter, Götz, Peter and Wolfgang at the beach in Zingst in 1940.

family traveled on holiday, although the boys continued to play in makeshift forts that they made near their home in Greiz.

Else sent food and gifts from the United States, wisely directing gifts to all four boys. Wolfgang recalled their excitement opening packages from Else. As a nine-year-old boy, Peter wrote the following to his mother (February 1940): "Liebe Mama, After a long break I am very happy for your letter dated January 15, today. And get the same day a chocolate gift from uncle Julie. For both I say my heartfelt thanks. You see, the latter was normal post and your letter, airmail, and what a tremendous difference lies in the travel duration. Yours, Peter."

By 1936, all children six years and older had to join a Nazi youth group. And so, shortly after arriving in Greiz at age six, Peter joined a Nazi youth group. At the younger age, the group focused on sports, hiking and camping to make it "fun" for young boys. At age 10, Peter was required to join *Jungvolk* (young people) and, at age 14, the boys were "promoted" to Hitler Youth. Peter dreaded the *Jungvolk* and Youth meetings. When he skipped meetings, as punishment he had to crawl "for hours" around the perimeter of a field, regardless of the weather. His communist friend also skipped meetings. Sometimes, they would crawl together and talk; they became good friends. At one of the *Jungvolk* meetings, when the group was soon to graduate to Hitler Youth, the boys were told "if anyone is unwilling to fight for their country, step forward." Everyone stood still, quiet. Peter's communist friend stepped forward, and Peter said, "somehow he lived." It was a dangerous thing to do, even as a young boy. You had to be careful what you said and did. One of the members of the local youth group reported that his father said "Hitler is an idiot," and his father was taken away by the authorities.

Food was rationed during the war. Peter, always hungry, told of once stealing bread from the slim shared family ration. His stepmother discovered his theft and scolded him. And, in response, Peter decided to get more food for the family by starting a garden and learning to bake. At 11 years old, he started growing potatoes and other vegetables. During his Greiz years he spent "all of his time" gardening and working on the farm of family friends in the summers to bring more food (including meat) into the household. Years later, as an adult in the United States, two of his favorite hobbies were gardening and baking.

Richard specialized in the chemistry of soaps and surfactants; his contributions to his field were documented in many patents both before and after the war. He was a lead chemist at Zschimmer and Schwarz in Greiz. As the years progressed into the 1940s, the chemical company in Greiz was taken over to aid the war effort. Albert Speer, the high-ranking Nazi party official and a Nuremberg trials criminal, was in charge of the chemists and physicists for the enforced generation of ammunition and war production.

During these years, Wolfgang described that the situation became increasingly tenuous for Richard. He led 200 workers at the chemical factory and his important leadership role protected him but also made him visible. His refusal to join the party and attend official meetings put him in danger. Richard hated the National Socialists and spoke openly within his family about his feelings. In 1933, the Nazis had issued a decree known as "For the Defense against Malicious Attacks against the Government," which required Germans to turn in anyone who spoke out against the party or its leaders. If the children spoke of their father's dissent, he would be put in a "KC" (concentration camp). It was particularly dangerous because Charlotte's father was an active Nazi and Richard at times argued with his father-in-law about the topic. Despite substantial pressure from his father-in-law, he continued to refuse to join the party. Charlotte pleaded with Richard to remain quiet.

Peter and his brothers remembered that Richard did many small things to prevent his sons from absorbing the nationalistic tendencies. For example, Richard had fenced in college and Peter was particularly interested in learning to fence, but fencing had come to be associated with nationalistic tendencies, "Deutschland über alles." When the boys expressed interest in fencing their father forbade it.

As the war progressed, younger children were recruited to fight, and Dieter was recruited before he turned 16. Richard tried to delay his deployment, and at first hid Dieter in their basement. But this became increasingly dangerous, as the penalty for avoiding service was execution by hanging. This was documented in a later family letter to Else, where Richard explained, "the penalty for such an offense was death" – hanging in the center of town – shortly before the end of the war, when they lived in Greiz. When Peter's "stepmother sent him into town he saw dead bodies of young men hanging in the center of town, and this made him very scared." So, at age 16, toward the end of the war, Dieter joined the anti-aircraft division, part of the German Air Force. His job was to "run" ammunitions for the Air Force. At the end of the war, as things became increasingly chaotic, Dieter deserted his military team and returned to live with his family in the countryside. In 1947, Richard wrote to Else about Dieter: "But you have to consider … that you are dealing with a person who at 16 years of age was put in with soldiers and even as a child had to deal with bombs."

The End of the War

The course of the war changed dramatically when Britain and the United States stormed Omaha Beach in Normandy, France, beginning to push the Nazis and their collaborators back. Dieter and Peter first heard about this June 6, 1944 event, "D-Day", listening to the BBC on Radio Europe. They had spent the months before learning English by regularly listening to the BBC. D-Day was codenamed Operation Overlord. Allied forces invaded with over 150,000 troops by air, ship and land. Dieter and Peter cheered; it was the beginning of the end of the war. However, the war, at that time, was still far from over.

In the following months, Richard knew that the war was almost over and that the Allied forces would soon be invading, bombing towns and cities across Germany, including Greiz. He took Peter and Dieter to see Dresden five months before the war ended. He wanted his sons to see the beautiful and ancient city of Dresden before it was bombed and destroyed, and indeed, at the end of the war, Dresden would be flattened.

Toward the end of the war, Richard had additional visits from the Nazis about joining the party and serving the war effort as a scientist. Richard continued to walk the fine line between doing his job and refusing to join the Nazi party despite significant pressure. Greiz was a likely target for Allied forces since it was home to a large chemical company in the neighboring valley, and hundreds of prisoners of war worked in forced labor in Sorgwald (near Thalbach, 2 km southeast of Greiz). In addition, the district hospital was a site where hundreds of people were forcibly sterilized by Nazis and where many chronically ill and elderly patients in care facilities were submitted to the euthanasia program "Aktion T4." As pressure increased, Richard hatched a scheme to placate the authorities and to get his family out of Greiz.

The story of how Richard moved the family to the country and bombed a hillside became family lore. Richard's scheme involved him convincing the Nazis that, as a chemist, he could generate a dynamite apparatus to "save" Germany, a type of "Copenhagen" bomb. To do this safely he would need to work in a remote farmhouse. One was chosen outside the small village of Neumühle, accessible to Greiz by small country trains that traveled through the woods. The officials agreed with his plan and gave him the dynamite to work on his war contraption. The family was moved to Neumühle for the months before the war ended. It was remote and safe, but there was also limited food available for the family. Peter walked from the farm, through the woods, to neighboring towns with a wheelbarrow, looking for food and supplies. As he traveled through the woods, Peter recalled seeing many German army deserters in tattered clothing and hungry, hiding in the woods.

Richard stored the dynamite in the basement of the farmhouse. As the Allied forces advanced, there was increasing bombing in the area. Richard realized that if the farmhouse was bombed, they would all certainly blow up because of all of the dynamite. He decided the dynamite had to be destroyed. He moved all of the explosives to a field far from the house and blew it up. The explosion was much larger than he expected, and it dug a large hole into the ground. It also caused all of the windows in the farmhouse to shatter. In the area at this time, there were many Russian and American soldiers roaming the region near Greiz. In this case, the American soldiers responded to the large explosion and came running across the field with their guns in hand. The children (Peter, his brothers and other farm children) were out in the field picking dandelions and were terrified as they watched the approaching American soldiers. Richard ran toward the children and the soldiers, and "miraculously" was able to speak fluent English to the soldiers. They had a friendly chat. He seemed to explain the situation to the Americans, who laughed and shook his hand jovially. The American soldiers smiled and gave the children chocolate candies. The children never knew exactly what their father said to the Americans.

Peter never spoke about what these explosives were actually used for, if anything. However, tales from family members after his death suggest that Dieter and Richard aided the Allied forces and set some of the explosives along rail lines that were used by the Nazis, to disable the tracks. At the end of the war, they blew up the explosives because they did not know if the Nazis, Russians or Americans would be the first to arrive at the farmhouse. Was Richard a "good" German? It is unclear if Richard had this kind of moral compass. However, one thing is clear. Somehow, despite significant pressure, he managed to both avoid joining the Nazi party and avoid getting into trouble with Nazi authorities. But even after the war, Richard's role during the war was not discussed. Even as a grandchild many years later, you knew not to ask this question.

In the later months of the war, Allied forces bombed Greiz but the damage was not extensive. The bombs destroyed the family garage and car, and heavily damaged the fields next to their home. Bombs largely destroyed Peter's school, as well as several bridges, but the old city center was largely spared. When the bombing ebbed and the Neumühle location became difficult to inhabit, the family moved back to their home in the Greiz. They found their home intact, but debris and bombs surrounded the area. Occasional lighter bombing also continued.

In order to stop the advance of the Americans, the Nazis systematically destroyed bridges. Some citizens in Greiz staged an uprising to block the Nazis and aid the advance of the Americans. A monument in Greiz recognizes an officer, Kurt von Westernhagen, who refused to follow Nazi orders to defend the town against the Allied forces and disbanded his soldiers. He took off his uniform and marched out of Greiz in support of Allied efforts. On his departure from Greiz the "deserter" von Westernhagen was shot and killed by the Gestapo, in April 1945.

After the War, Greiz in the Russian Zone

Peter was 14 years old in 1945. Their house, Clos Strasse 13 in Greiz, had been spared. Their garage was bombed, the fields next to their home were bombed, their school was bombed. In the days and months after the war moved beyond Greiz, the kids continued to play, as kids do, in the areas littered with rubble.

The family was hopeful. The Americans were now in charge. The war was ending. It was a time for celebration! But then the Russian soldiers moved in. Saxonia and Turin became part of the Soviet zone.

The change was fast. In 1945, the Russians started gathering German scientists to move them to the Soviet Union. Richard managed to be one step ahead. One night, with no warning to his children, Richard fled to the west alone, by freight train. Peter later learned that, in the middle of the night, Russian soldiers would arrive with machine guns and take scientists away – to Siberia or other areas of the Soviet Union. As the Russian initiative became more organized it was referred to as Operation Osoaviakhim. A few thousand scientists and their families were moved from the eastern occupied zones of Germany to the Soviet Union. The plan was to have them work as scientists for the Russians. But at the time, what Peter knew was that his father had left his family behind.

Richard traveled by freight train to Braubach, a small village along the Rhine in the west of Germany, close to where they had lived before the war.

He hoped to find a job again at Zschimmer and Schwarz, his former chemical company near Lahnstein. Dieter, and then Peter, uncertain and eager to reunite with their father, wrote letters in November 1945. First from Dieter:

Dear Father,

Now that it is allowed to write letters, I would like to use this Sunday to write you. Hopefully you can read because I am only allowed to write in Latin language – and it is difficult for me. We just came back from our Sunday afternoon walk through the park and back home. Everyone sits around the dinner table – mom is knitting, Wolfi makes homework and Peter helps him. And Götz sits on his chair and looks at picture books. We are all still healthy and even the food is good. Nobody is leaving the table hungry but everyone has to work for the food. Mother is driving to Russeldorf and Peter goes in the countryside scavenging for food. And Wolfi is collecting horse manure so next year we have more in our garden. I still go to Ritters and I don't know any more how our house looks at daylight. In the morning I leave in the dark and I return in the dark. In our room lives now a married couple and mother does not like it when she comes in the kitchen and listens to the complaints of the couple. Thank God they are looking for a different apartment because we don't help them enough, and they are "poor refugees." They are leaving because we are not helpful to the "poor" refugee. If everyone would be as rich as they are none of us would be in trouble. Everywhere we notice your absence and particularly on Sundays we think about you – and the whole day we say how nice it would be if dad were here to eat with us. Now I will finish in hopes of seeing you soon.

Peter wrote:

Dear father

Hopefully you will soon visit us because we miss you everywhere. Wolfi told me to tell you to come soon because a screw broke on his bicycle. Please write us soon. We are healthy; only mom was not feeling too well yesterday. Maybe because Frau Lindemann (the "refugee") was the whole day in the kitchen. Herr Oberst comes in and reads the newspaper "how one should treat the poor refugees" – I feel really sick from it. My school started one week ago but we have it only 3 days per week and they dismissed almost all of the teachers. It costs 300 Marks per year. We still scavenge potatoes and I went a few times to Dobia and I found some food there. Hopefully we hear from you soon.

The refugees were part of a large exodus of Germans who were expelled from Poland and Hungary. They moved in with German families in the eastern zone, and there was no choice but to host these refugees in the months after the war ended.

After there was no word from Richard, Dieter decided to leave in search of their father. He traveled to Braubach, by freight train. At age 14, Peter for the first time was left without his mother Else, father Richard or brother Dieter. It had been a long time since they had last seen or heard from their father. It was not clear if he would return, or if they would see him again. Peter's stepmother Charlotte was lonely and scared, and was also increasingly absent. Peter was often left alone to take care of his younger brothers. Wolfgang recalled at that time receiving a bad head injury, which left a scar on his forehead. Peter was alone with the boys and took care of him, cleaning and bandaging his wound. As Wolfgang later said, "Peter always helped me." This caregiving role likely contributed to his later interest in becoming a physician who cared for children.

Peter had a strained relationship with his stepmother at that time. He did not trust her and felt he needed to know where she was going, in case he needed her help. So, on one of her outings, he followed her and discovered a secret tryst. He hid and watched until she emerged from the house. Maybe she knew he was watching. Peter thought his stepmother never liked him, except for the gardening:

December 12, 1945

Dear Father

Your letter to Dieter and me arrived earlier this week and thank you. I hope Dieter arrived safely at your place. Since he will be with you, I hope you will not be lonely. Last day of school – Christmas holiday until January 3. We now have the old subjects except history and geography. Russian is now taught starting in 6th grade. Now we have all 9 grades. In the garden we have a good harvest; mostly pears abundant on our tree. I think more than last year. Also, *Spätkraut* (cabbage) was plentiful. We even have enough to make sauerkraut. We have red beets. The carrots we put in a sandbox in the basement. I asked the house manager if we will have more storage next year. The man was very angry and said it was due to the communists. But now here, it is good to be a communist.

Wolfi was also helpful and he collected horse manure which I will put on the strawberries and make sure we will have a double harvest next year. I already prepared the garden. We cannot get cow manure. We have enough potatoes and you do not need to be worried about us. We got our winter

potatoes and this will be enough for us for the winter. Unfortunately, they were not as good as last year's potatoes. I went to Dobia because it was the farthest away from the city. I hid some of the food away in the country. The toy village that I built for Götz was completed; for Wolfi I built a bird house but it is not completed. It is not so shabby as the one we built a few years ago. In addition to glue, I also nailed it together. We don't have any winter weather and the last days were very warm.
I wish you a nice Christmas. And best regards from your
Peter

In 1946, the conditions in Greiz deteriorated. Movement also became more difficult, and Russian enforcement increased. Charlotte decided it was time to try to flee to the west to join Richard and Dieter. Travel with children was difficult. Peter was 14, Wolfgang was 8, and Götz was 6 years old. The countryside near Greiz was littered with debris and fleeing people. Bridges had been destroyed and roads were often impassable. Charlotte arranged their night passage on a freight train, in exchange for their car. They drove in darkness to the train, with the headlights off, and turned over the keys to the car. At the train they joined other people also fleeing to the west. Before they were allowed in the cattle car, they all had to strip down, including Charlotte, and were sprayed with disinfectant for delousing. They tried to sleep on the hard floor of the cattle car, crowded with other people all fleeing to the west. It was a tough trip but timely because they fled, as Wolfgang later put it, two years before the "metal" between the east and west was erected and it became nearly impossible to leave the east. They had made it out of the Soviet zone.

6 IN BRAUBACH, AFTER THE WAR

In 1946, Peter's family reunited in Braubach, a village along the Rhine near Koblenz and Oberlahnstein, Peter's birthplace. Braubach is a medieval village lined with half-timbered buildings that run along narrow winding streets. Nestled in the hills along the Rhine, Braubach is surrounded by vineyards and forest, and was left largely intact after the war. From all points in town including the Marktplatz (marketplace in the town center), the Marksburg castle is visible on the hill above the village. Initially constructed in the 1100s, the castle was badly damaged during the war and was left in ruins for years. During Peter's teenage years, the castle served as an adventure playground for the youth of Braubach. However, in current times the Marksburg castle has been restored and is now part of the Rhine Gorge UNESCO World Heritage Sites. The family lived in a small apartment near the town center, Rhinestrasse 3. Peter and Dieter shared a room with a window that had a view of the castle.

In 1945, Richard returned to Zschimmer und Schwarz in Lahnstein to find that there was no permanent work. This made it difficult to have his family join him since there were limited resources or food for a family of six. Richard had attempted to transfer his car from Greiz to Braubach because he realized the substantial value of a vehicle at that time and the importance of having one to find food. He had his car dismantled in Greiz and shipped to Zschimmer and Schwarz in Lahnstein. A French army officer in Lahnstein intercepted the shipment and had the car rebuilt. The officer, an inexperienced driver, attempted to drive the car only to smash it into a tree, demolishing it. Richard was left with no car and no other options for cars in Braubach. The car was one of Richards strategies for "making it for his family" after the war, but it was not to be.

Needing to be resourceful, Richard instead started a medicinal chemistry operation from the cellar of his apartment building. Before the arrival of his family, Richard arranged housing with Dr. Deutsch, a renegade physician in Braubach whom he had known from before the war. Richard collaborated with Dr. Deutsch to start a chemical fabrication business to manufacture laxatives and other health remedies in exchange for food and other provisions from local farmers.

Wolfgang described the post-war years: "We were all hungry. Peter and Dieter distributed the medicine products to the farmers by bicycle, in exchange for food. They also worked in the vineyards all seasons. This is how the family survived and fed four growing boys." Peter also developed a close friendship with the baker next to their home. Peter would help him, in exchange for some bread, further contributing to his lifelong love of baking.

Richard wrote the following letter to Else:

December 8, 1946

Dear Else!

The letters of the boys tell you how it is with us. It is modest in every respect, but we must not let our heads hang down and must try to get through this time of misery with our skins intact. I don't know if we can get our furniture and household goods out of the east. But I would rather be here without furniture than to disappear with the family somewhere in Russia, like so many colleagues. I wish you a very blessed and happy Christmas and with best wishes for the New Year. I greet you also in the name of my wife. I celebrated your birthday with the boys while chopping wood in the forest!

As your, Richard

Scavenging for food continued to be Peter's focus after the war in Braubach. Wolfgang and Peter searched for mushrooms in the forest near the castle ruins, and close to their home. One month, they came upon the largest mushrooms they had ever seen. No other families were gathering mushrooms at the time because several families had become ill and a whole family had died eating white mushrooms from the same woods. Wolfgang said, "Peter was very good at identifying edible mushrooms," an early sign of Peter's observational skills and interest in biology. Wolfgang relished telling how they gathered many mushrooms in the forest and this made for "delicious" family meals for weeks.

After the war, Else started in earnest to arrange the transit of Peter and Dieter to America. Richard wrote a candid letter to Else in December 1947, concerning the difficult decision to send his boys to America. The translated letter is quoted in full as a remarkable window into that time and place.

Dear Else,

Your letter of the 4th of this month has triggered a tremendous excitement and great consultations and discussions here. The fact that Peter is going to leave us as well is a bit too much at once and a proposal that we must first process. Besides, I am worried whether you won't be frightened by how the boys will break into your peace and turn your house upside down, so that after 8 days you will have to buy them a ticket back to Europe.

In any case, I thank you in the name of the boys for this invitation. As difficult as it is for us to give them away, this consideration should not play a role in the decision, since the happiness and developmental potential of the children should be the sole deciding factor. We also hope that they will settle in the new country and that they will bring not merely care and trouble but also joy into your home. Coincidently, I just found out that it's not possible to emigrate from the French occupation zone to other countries except France. I have tried to register Dieter and Peter in Stuttgart. They will be registered pro forma in Stuttgart, Alte Weinsteige 20, and Dieter will smuggle himself to Stuttgart next week to have issued the registration papers and identity cards for himself and Peter. Things are not that easy anymore and there are different laws and regulations in every zone and every occupying power takes care of its sheep differently. On the way back from Stuttgart, Dieter is supposed to go to the consulate in Frankfurt to see if the papers have arrived yet. Then I will go to the American consul myself so that the applications will not remain in the queue forever.

Then I inquired whether the passage from here could be paid in Reichsmark but got a negative answer from two offices in Stuttgart and Cologne. Germans are not allowed to own and buy foreign currency and the passages are only noted in dollars, guilders or pounds. But I will also inquire directly in Hamburg and Bremen because all travel agencies make a rather disoriented impression; it hardly ever happens that someone from here wants to make an overseas trip these days.

On Sunday I was in Stuttgart at Grandma's birthday, and I found her quite lively, although she has become quite old and shaky. The house in the Weinsteige is now from top to bottom crowded with lodgers and I just found a small sofa in a room on which I could stretch my bones. The lowest floor is occupied by a family and upstairs the rooms are also occupied by two lodgers. But at least the house is habitable again and the roof is closed again, so that Grandma has a place to stay for her old age. I told her, too, that you invited the boys to visit you. And she, too, as hard as it is for her to give them up, since she will not be able to see them anymore, she wants that they have the opportunity to get out of Germany. She sends her best regards to you, dear Else, and asks you to see to it that the two become good and righteous men who stand their ground in life. She can't write to you herself because her hands have become too shaky, and I had to promise her that I would write to you on her behalf. You know how attached she is to the children and how dear they are to her heart! And she still thinks that we, the young, don't do it right if we don't accept her advice. But the young have already become older men with gray hair who should actually know themselves what's necessary. Fritz has also put in his two cents about the boys' big trip and, as a real professor, has brought descriptions and maps of Buffalo and the surrounding towns so that Dieter can get his bearings. Fritz, by the way, looks quite bad and old because his stay as a *möblierter Herr* (furnished gentleman) in Tübingen has taken quite a lot out of him and after the life in Tübingen during weekdays he comes to Stuttgart on Friday evening, completely exhausted and starved, to feed himself over the weekend. I didn't go to Jule's because time was quite short, and Dieter will visit him in the next few days when he will come to Stuttgart. I wanted to buy an etching showing the view from Olgastr. to the Stiftskirche after the destruction of Stuttgart: but it was not for sale and Trude will now try to find something similar so that you can picture your hometown as it looks today, although it is better not to see it and not to destroy the images of your memory.

Our life here has become more difficult in recent months, as the hardship has taken on almost unimaginable forms. How we can get through this winter with the allotment of one hundredweight of potatoes and with the miniature rations is a mystery to me at the moment. In Rhineland-Palatinate we received not even one gram of meat in November and today, for the first time, 75 grams of fat. At the same time, we have to watch how freight trains full of wine and butter go west every day, while here the population is literally starving. Hopefully, the London conference will bring an end to this exploitation, which is unbearable in the long run. The French have not only failed to seize their great chance to take the lead on the European continent but have only made enemies and evoked hatred everywhere.

I had a lot of sympathy for France, but I have changed my mind due to this corruption and exploitation economy and I have seen that their methods of plundering are even superior to those of Hitler. With little skill and diplomacy, they could have easily created a union of nations in Europe, which would perhaps have given the old continent a different face in a few years. And I am afraid that all the credits that Europe has received under this leadership are wasted and can just as well be thrown into the sea because they are squandered away by France just like all previous credits. That's why I am so pessimistic and fear that in a few years Stalin will be hailed and longed for as triumphator everywhere in Europe because his European counterparts are so inept and short-sighted that all the cards will be taken out of their hands.

And since I consider this political development unstoppable, if the USA does not directly dictate the political direction and leadership on the European continent, I am particularly glad that Dieter and Peter will escape this chaos here. Because I don't think it is opportune that the boys will be here and possibly have to fight for Stalin against America. But all this would be different, if the European West would get together and take the necessary steps today, knowing the danger coming from the East. And the most important step is to stabilize the economy and life again and to oppose the communist propaganda with the prosperity and the power of the democratic states.

But we are not being listened to and at the moment we are the object that is being plundered by France and Russia. It is grotesque when the small French occupation zone exported to France for 11.2 billion francs in 1946, while old Germany exported 11.6 billion francs in 1938. The small zone with 5.6 million inhabitants has to raise as much as formerly the whole German Reich. According to official Paris statistics, France shipped 2 billion francs worth of goods to the occupied zone in 1946, mainly old, spoiled potatoes and other goods that could not be sold on the market. In addition, there were large exports that went illegally to France through the smuggling of the occupation forces, which accounted for billions. This is the balance sheet of a supposedly cultural nation and a country that claims to carry the flag of democracy and human rights. Whereas, when seen correctly, they are just as miserable street robbers as the representatives of the Third Reich.

But we keep carrying our heads upright and will bounce back. However, I do not believe in a recovery of Europe if there won't come a strong hand from somewhere else that brings order into this stable. As sad as this conclusion is, it really seems that Europe, with the exception of the Russians, has run down and no longer has the strength to renew itself. And given this outlook I am glad that you want to help the boys, and that they are at least out of Europe until one gets an idea of how everything will turn out. Therefore, I thank you once again for all that you are willing to do for the sake of the boys and I hope and wish that this step will lead them to a better future. With best greetings from house to house.

I am always yours,
Richard

This was the reality of Peter's teenage years. Little did Richard or his sons know at the time that, as Richard had hoped, the Americans would soon answer the call to leadership in the democratic west. Beginning in 1948, the United States implemented the Marshall Plan, a bold effort to improve the economy of western Europe and boost the fortunes of a new Germany. Richard could not have known when he wrote his letter that such relief would be forthcoming or how incredibly successful the Marshall Plan would be, impacting the daily lives of Germans in 1948 but also the shape of European and global politics for decades to come.

In a later follow-up letter in 1949 Richard continued his discussion:

And have you ever considered that the burdens imposed on us by the occupying armies are greater than what the Marshall Plan has given us? If Germany had not been robbed and plundered in such a senseless way, the American and British taxpayers wouldn't have to pay for saving us Germans from naked starvation. This excursion into politics was necessary to help you understand the boys.

Braubach was in the French zone. Richard described the post-war conditions in another letter to Else, further explaining what Peter and Dieter had experienced:

In the east where the Russians, who were worse than animals – and even in the west – French divisions moved in to free southern Germans in a way that all women and girls were abused. They stole and destroyed everything in the name of freedom and democracy – and although they have gotten better this process still has not finished. You know I was very sympathetic to France before – and I was always taking their part – and I would always help a French prisoner in any way that was in my control. And how did I get to know this grand nation after the war? – they were called the west Russians by the Germans. That seems to hit the nail on the head. To this day, one would never have thought this was possible of this cultured nation. I still recognize now as before the intellectual capabilities of France – because I knew them before and learned to appreciate them. But how difficult it is for a young person who knows nothing else but being badly treated by them.

And in another letter Richard wrote:

You must keep in mind that the boys were brought up in the spirit of constant rejection and criticism of Nazism. But after we finally got rid of the Nazis, the hell really got started for us. In the East, the Russians acted worse than animals, and even in the West, French divisions arrived as "liberators" while raping women and girls all over southern Germany. In addition, robbery and plunder took place in the name of freedom and democracy, and this process has not yet found an end, even if it's conducted in a somewhat refined form. Hundreds of thousands of people met a horrible end in the German concentration camps. But we always had to reckon with the fact that we might be next because giving a cigarette to a foreign prisoner or a Jew was enough to make us disappear in a concentration camp. But after the end of the war, when we were all waiting for the return of humane conditions, millions of the most innocent women and children were murdered in Russia, Poland and the Czech Republic, millions starved to death in the most horrible way in Germany. Those whom we had joyfully expected as our liberators from the Nazi yoke behaved like Hitler's brutal henchmen. These experiences have made the boys skeptical and oversensitive.

The boys attended school part – time during these years. The *Gymnasium* was in Lahnstein and had been bombed. Peter went to school in the cellar of the ruins remaining from the former school in Lahnstein. Wolfgang attended the same *Gymnasium* six years later in the basement, with the same Latin teacher, who had lost his arm in the war. The time was bad. Germany was a "destroyed land." Richard could not find permanent work in the Lahnstein area and, due to a growing conflict with Dr. Deutsch, Richard started to look for new opportunities. It was difficult to feed his family without reliable work.

During this time, care packages from Else in the United States continued to help the family. Wolfgang remembered looking forward to these care packages from Else, because he was always "hungry." In addition to food, Else also sent treats of cocoa and gifts for the four boys. Around this time, Richard and Else started the long process of trying to move Dieter and Peter to the United States. It had always been the intention for Else to reunite with her boys when the war ended and conditions stabilized. However, it was difficult to persuade the Americans initially to take young German men, especially Dieter, who had served in the German army. The following letter is from Peter to Else, dated January 1948:

Dear Mom,

I thank you for your Christmas package – everything that you sent was perfect.

We have had so little to eat, and the two little ones [Wolfgang and Götz] were very happy with their part of the package – there was big excitement at New Year's Eve and for the party.

On New Year's Day the weather was so beautiful – as it has not been since 1926. The weather now is terrible here. It has been raining and you don't notice very much about winter. I had a lot of fun for many hours because we were under water – it appeared almost as if we were in Venice. We needed a new house door because of the flooding. We are unable to ski. We would have to be in St. Moritz where we could watch the Olympics. I have finished the school semester satisfactorily but we are getting less and less schooling as the cultural and the economic position of Germany is soon going to collapse. On some days we have only three classes so it is hardly worthwhile traveling there. We have biology and geography. Music and arithmetic do not exist anymore. It is totally unimportant. But we get quite a lot of homework so that we are up to all hours of the night doing work. The reports are getting worse and worse so it cannot go on much longer. Except for the German oil we have not received anything for 3 months but there are some countries that still believe that the Germans are still doing too well. It would be to their advantage if they got to know us more harmoniously so that they could be cured of their impressions. We have not heard yet about the exact date of our leaving – it will be quite a while before we hear about this –

I hope everything is ok.

I wish you the best greetings and a big kiss
Peter

In the months before leaving Germany in 1948, Peter wrote to Else:

Dear Mom,

I was very pleased with the shirt and the pajamas and the sweets. They also tasted very good. I also thank you very much for the last letter – only a pity that you are still ill. I wish you a speedy recovery so that for Easter you will be well and happy and can celebrate it. Since Dieter wrote, a care package has also arrived for which I thank you very much. Because of that we can actually bake a real cake for Easter. Last week Dieter and I were asked to go see immigration officials. We were interrogated by an American officer and examined about our political views. The officer was, by the way, the first man I have met who was actually polite to Germans. The others seem to believe that they have to appear rough. When he heard that Dieter served in the Airforce he shook his head somewhat doubtfully and threw us a dubious look. We could not find out from him whether there was a possibility for Dieter to get what we were asking for – he would not help us. We simply have to hope and wait. We were told that we would hear in around 3 months. I would really not like to travel alone. I have to ask you something else – in school in the last few weeks we were able to read American papers – amongst them the *New York Times*. I was a little bit surprised how they talked about whether you have done something and how you need to own up to it. When you read this – you could soon assume that America was already prepared for another war – and that it would be totally willing to enter into another war. Write to me and tell me if this is true and the view of the majority of the American people – I hope not.

Soon I will write a letter to you in English. Today I do not feel in the mood to do it as there is beautiful weather outside and I would prefer to go out for a while. At last, the sun is shining after many foggy typical winter days. The sun is really shining. To add to this, soon we have Easter holidays and more I can't ask for – to have holidays when the sun is shining. If it is going to be as beautiful at Easter, I want to take a hike with my friends, probably on Easter Monday. I went to a concert in Koblenz – to a Beethoven performance – I totally loved it. I still believe I have never heard more beautiful music before. If only you could hear something like this more often. Now I will stop. Once again I hope you feel better soon.

With hearty greetings to uncle Max. I am also enclosing one of the many pictures I had to take for my immigration papers.

Peter

[Note from Peter to Else's husband Max:]

Thank you for what you are doing for us and making it possible for us to come to America. For you I am sure it is a difficult decision to want to take us in. I hope we will make it up to you.

Later, as an adult, Peter would agree that all of the above was true, but would reliably mention that their lives at the time were not all gloom. Despite the difficult post-war conditions Peter did find opportunities for fun, such as hiking and rock climbing with his friends (Figure 6.1).

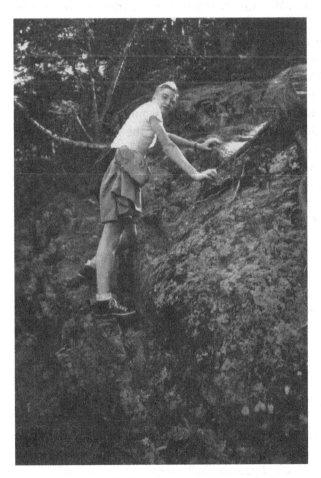

Figure 6.1 Peter rock climbing in the hills near Braubach, in the French District of Germany, after the war.

7 ARRIVAL IN AMERICA

Peter and Dieter traveled to "America" on the *Marine Shark*, a US cargo ship (Figure 7.1). The trip, as Peter understood it, was to "visit their mother." Peter had not seen his mother since he was six years old. Intermittent letters and the packages of food and gifts were the only contacts. Peter refused to make the trip without Dieter, whose approval by the US government was delayed because he had helped in the German Airforce. Richard and Charlotte prepared Dieter and Peter for their transit, putting together a photo album for the boys with childhood photos. Dieter and Peter arrived in Ellis Island at the end of 1948, shortly before Peter's 18th birthday (Figure 7.2).

When Else and Richard had agreed years earlier that the boys would at some point reunite with their mother, no one realized this would take over a decade. Else and Richard both thought the opportunities for the boys in the United States were better than in Germany. By 1948 Else was particularly eager to get the boys to the United States because they were listed as dependents on her naturalization papers and US citizenship would be "automatic" for them if they resided in the United States as minors.

In a letter from Richard to Else in 1949, he wrote:

Thank you for the letters. They gave me a clear impression of the development of both boys in their new home because you can imagine that I have great worries about them and how they find their way and if they have the right relationship with you and your new husband. Both of them are really out of their impressionable age and can be regarded as adults. Both come from a country where youth was torn apart and they were very skeptical towards the rest of the world. Let the boys find their peace – and let them find their way to separate themselves from their past. Until now this is what had impressed their young lives. I am quite sure Dieter will get this understanding once he settles in the United States. And that the democratic freedom does not have to be expressed in bad behavior such as cigarette smoking but he can pursue intellectual work and be imaginative – if he wants to do it. He is an active football player – but I would not be in favor of him ignoring English and chemical studies and takes football instead.

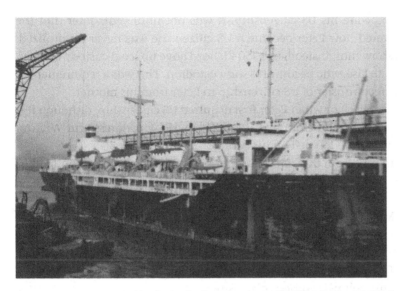

Figure 7.1 Peter arrived in the United States through Ellis Island with his brother Dieter on the SS *Marine Shark*, a cargo ship built by the US Maritime.

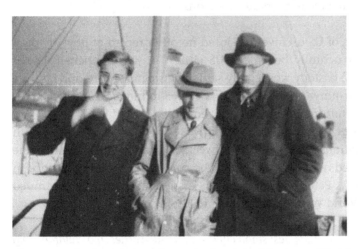

Figure 7.2 The first picture of Peter in the United States, at Ellis Island with his brother and unknown man, shortly after meeting his mother for the first time since he was six years old.

Peter arrived in the United States and immediately enrolled in Lafayette High School in Buffalo, to learn English and complete his final semester of high school before attending university. Unbeknownst to Peter, his parents were working to expedite his US citizenship. It was not until years later that the family discovered how Peter became a US citizen. He was never naturalized. Documents show that, instead, in 1950 Richard gave up legal custody of Peter, then aged 19, to Else, who became his sole custodian. This was a requirement to enable the direct transfer of US citizenship to Peter from his mother.

It is not entirely clear when Peter first acquired US citizenship, although it is certain that it occurred before he turned 21. In 1950, congressman William l. Pfeifer from Buffalo lobbied on his behalf.

A telegram sent from the office of immigration to the congressman read as follows:

> May 16 1950. Radiogram to your office. Staff recom-
> mendations favorable. Family is anxious for
> a college scholarship.
> Telegram: recommendation favorable.
> Through his mother: sole custody.
> Police record in Germany: no record
> Emigration services: no record of naturalization
> Certificate: recommendation favorable.

Extensive searching of US archives disclosed no other record of how or when Peter Huttenlocher actually became a US citizen. It just happened. Dieter turned 21 before the custody was legally settled between Richard and Else. He would return to Germany briefly, but then decided to make the United States his home, and was naturalized as a US citizen later.

For young men at that time, citizenship was very much a matter of both benefits and obligations. In later letters between Else and Richard, Else became increasingly agitated about the boys and the compulsory military service in the United States. As Peter predicted, the US engagement in wars continued after the Second World War. Richard wrote to Else:

> *Thus, the old saying still applies: small children – small worries, big children – big worries! Hopefully they do not burden you too much and you can cope with them, provided that the American military service does not put a spoke in your wheel. This is a looming specter for me, too. I had not reckoned with the possibility that the boys would be called up for military service before naturalization. It would certainly be a catastrophe. But let's wait and see. They still have the possibility to come back here if the draft cannot be averted otherwise.*

The University of Buffalo: Discovering Philosophy – and a Life Partner

Peter had arrived in the United States at age 17 and, for the first time, lived with his mother (endearingly called "moo coo" by Peter and Dieter) and his step-father Max. He continued to live with them when he enrolled the following fall at the University of Buffalo. He studied philosophy and pre-medicine. Peter was grateful to Else and Max for taking them in and family members later remembered that he embarked on being good: a good person, a good student and good at whatever he was doing. He was no longer in a post-war country and the early 1950s was a time of prosperity and hope in the United States.

Peter's first close friend in the United States was Joel Spiegelman. They met in summer school organic chemistry, several months after Peter's arrival in the country. Joel, the son of Russian Jewish immigrants, was bold and "pretty radical" as a student at the University of Buffalo. After flailing through summer chemistry, Joel went on to become a talented composer, conductor and harpsichord performer both in the United States and Russia, and Peter's life-long friend.

In an interview in March 2019, Joel described Peter when they met. He was a "blond guy with an accent, from Koblenz, very nice; his English was ok; we shared an interest in music and philosophy. . . . [He told me how] his home was bombed; otherwise, he was a fresh immigrant and did not talk about it." Joel immediately liked Peter. He had a strong "sense of inquiry and curiosity." Joel also said: "I could say anything to Peter; you do not have many friendships like that in a lifetime."

Joel further recalled: "Our culture was different, but we shared music and left-wing politics; we both wanted to change the world." During their college years, they took philosophy together and attended basement anti-Stalin meetings. Peter attended an international Trotsky meeting in Buffalo with Joel to learn more about Trotskyism, a variant of Marxism. From his year living in the Russian zone, Peter was anti-Stalin. Joel was also anti-Stalin and, as Joel said, in those years he was "pretty radical." Indeed, Joel's college "activities" earned him an interview with the CIA (Central Intelligence Agency).

Both Peter and Joel were heavily influenced by their philosophy professor and chair of the Department of Philosophy at the University of Buffalo, Dr. Marvin Farber. Interestingly, his brother, Sidney Farber, was a famous cancer researcher at Harvard Medical School and the namesake of the Farber Cancer Institute in Boston. It is likely that both Peter's strong academic performance at the University of Buffalo and this connection with Sidney Farber later helped Peter gain acceptance to Harvard Medical School.

Marvin Farber was an influential philosopher, the founder and long-time editor of the journal *Philosophy and Phenomenological Research*, and is credited with introducing phenomenology to the United States. For a young man who had grown up with Nazism and lived in the Soviet and French occupied zone of Germany as Peter did, it was easy to become fascinated with phenomenology, the philosophy of experience. What is human consciousness and imagination? What is the situation of humans in society and history? How do you investigate phenomena as consciously experienced? It is hard for us to understand how a child consciously experiences a childhood in war and Nazism. What are the memories or imagined experiences that evolved from what Peter lived through as a child? The concepts of memory, consciousness and experience consumed Peter's thinking at the time. This kind of thinking and immersion in philosophy helped to drive his future interests in understanding the development of the human brain.

During his immersion in philosophy and American college life Peter met his future wife, Janellen, in a philosophy seminar at the University of Buffalo. Joel knew "Jane" Burns from their grade school piano class. Jane also grew up in an eastern European immigrant family of Jewish descent. Her family never owned a house or a car, and she was determined to do well in school and grow up to live in one of the "nice old houses" in the wealthy neighborhood near her family's rental apartment in Buffalo. At the start of university, Jane changed her name from Jane to Janellen, combining her first and middle names, because Jane seemed too "plain." Janellen's father Alan was one of 10 children and had to leave school at the age of 10 to work in a factory to help support his family after his father abandoned them. Alan, like Richard, had a knack for chemistry. Janellen recalled him experimenting with chemicals in the attic of their apartment building when she was a child, to make tanning lotion to sell for extra money during the depression. Janellen's father worked as a linotype operator to print newspapers and lost his job during the depression. Unlike Richard, he did not have formal training as a chemist. One of his chemistry experiments caused an explosion in the attic of their apartment and the roof was demolished and had to be replaced. As Janellen tells it, "my father lost his hair in the explosion and it never grew back." Janellen's mother also came from an immigrant family; her mother's father was a charismatic union organizer after immigrating to the United States. Janellen adored her maternal grandmother, her Oma, who had a thick German accent and cooked potato latkes and served German kuchen. She was from the borderlands of eastern Europe where people spoke both Yiddish and German. It was therefore not a surprise that Janellen immediately liked Peter and was intrigued by his accent and background.

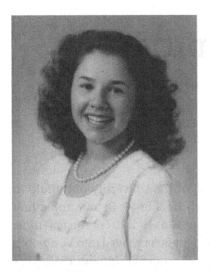

Figure 7.3 Photo of Jane Burns, later Janellen Huttenlocher, as a teenager.

Janellen was chatty, an avid reader and smart as a whip. As a former teenage "beauty queen," Janellen commanded Peter's attention and interest (Figure 7.3). Janellen reported with a smile: "Suddenly Peter was there by my side – talking to me and following me around." Peter invited Janellen for dinner at Joel's apartment, to "talk about philosophy." He was "gracious and lovely; he liked to talk about reality and philosophy." They all started to gather at a coffee place near campus – "a nickel a cup" – and sit for hours with friends, talking about philosophy and ideas. Janellen said that Peter "was interested in what made people good, in how to be good, and thought that one could only be happy if one was good to others." Then they would go to a nearby hot-dog stand on the edge of Buffalo and have "hot dogs with everything on them – always burned – grilled and delicious." Joel, his girlfriend Gail, Janellen and Peter would venture out in Joel's convertible and go to Crystal Beach in Canada, on the other side of the Peace Bridge. On one occasion, when Peter and Janellen were at a pizza parlor in a rough neighborhood, a group of thugs approached Janellen and said "get the girl." Peter tried to reason with the thugs, but when one of them grabbed Janellen, the gentle and calm Peter responded with a swift left-handed punch. The surprised thugs fled. It turns out that Peter had learned to defend himself as a teenager in the Soviet and French post-war occupation zones. After this encounter Janellen knew that Peter was the guy for her, and that he would take good care of her. Years later, Janellen loved to tell the story about Peter and his left-handed punch.

8 HARVARD MEDICAL SCHOOL

After completing his undergraduate training at the University of Buffalo in three years, Peter started at Harvard Medical School in 1953, four and a half years after arriving in the United States through Ellis Island. For the first time, Peter was really on his own. As a first-year student Peter moved into Vanderbilt Hall, a dormitory for male Harvard medical students. In the 1950s, the Harvard medical class was largely composed of elite highly educated men, many of whom had attended Harvard College or other Ivy League institutions. By living in Vanderbilt, Peter became fully immersed in an entirely new culture of the American elite.

How did a young German man come to be accepted into Harvard in the early 1950s? As previously noted, Peter credited his acceptance in part to the connection between his philosophy professor at the University of Buffalo, Marvin Farber, and Marvin's brother Sidney Farber, a medical school professor at Harvard and namesake for the future Farber Cancer Institute. But Peter was also a star student and a favorite of Marvin Farber, who shared his interests in human motivation. By the time Peter started medical school his English was fluent, but he continued to speak with a thick German accent throughout his life. In these early years in the United States, Peter was sometimes taunted and called a "Nazi." In subsequent years, when asked where he was from, he would often say "Buffalo, NY." When people looked at him askew, he smiled. It was not always popular to be German in the United States in the 1950s.

During medical school Peter worked particularly hard. He wanted to make up for the gaps in his own education, and he was also interested in what he was learning. The first-year students spent hours in the basement of one of the large marble-faced buildings on the medical school quadrangle at Harvard, learning anatomy. Working in teams of four students, they spent grueling hours dissecting a human cadaver in a room effused with the smell of formaldehyde. For the first time, Peter had an intimate glimpse into the workings of the human body and the nervous system. Hours were spent dissecting the many

interconnected nerves and muscles of the human body and memorizing the anatomical names in Latin. His Latin class with the one-armed teacher in the bombed-out basement of his high school in Lahnstein served him well.

A rite of passage for Harvard medical students was attending lectures in the iconic Ether Dome in Massachusetts General Hospital. Medical students and physicians in training listened to lectures in this amphitheatre with an operating stage below in the center of the dome. The Ether Dome was first built as an operating amphitheatre in 1821, and students and trainees would watch "brutal" surgeries performed on conscious patients since there was no effective anesthesia. On "Ether Day," October 16, 1846, the first public demonstration of the use of inhaled ether as a surgical anesthetic took place in the Ether Dome, launching modern-day anesthesiology. The first patient to receive ether, Gilbert Abbott, awoke from neck surgery with no pain or memory of the surgery, and said it felt like a "scratch" on his neck.

In addition to his classroom studies, Peter delved into fundamental research in the first year of medical school under the guidance of the German pharmacologist Otto Krayer. Peter had met Krayer during his medical-school interview, and Krayer took an immediate interest in Peter and his history. Dr. Krayer had a history that was similar to Peter's mother Else and this led to an immediate understanding and connection. Krayer had risked speaking up because, according to Avram Goldstein's biographical memoir published in 1987, he "believed, very simply, that a person had to do what their conscience said was right, that in such matters it was not a question of weighing consequences" [1]. Krayer was a talented young scientist in Germany in 1932 when he was offered a chair position at a University in Dusseldorf. When he learned that the university offered this position because they had relieved a Jewish professor of the position, Krayer refused to accept the appointment. He wrote to the officials, "the primary reason for my reluctance is that I feel the exclusion of Jewish scientists to be an injustice, the necessity of which I cannot understand, since it has been justified by reasons that lie outside the domain of science. This feeling of injustice is an ethical phenomenon. It is innate to the structure of my personality, and not something imposed from the outside." In response to being told he had to accept the position, he refused. The following was the official response from the Prussian Minister for Science, Art and National Education [1, p. 151]:

In your letter of 15 June, you state that you feel the barring of Jewish scientists is an injustice, and that your feelings about this injustice prevent you from accepting a position offered to you. You are of course personally free to feel any way you like about the way the government acts. It is not acceptable, however, for you to make the practice of your teaching profession dependent upon those feelings. You would

in that case not be able in the future to hold any chair in a German university.
Pending final decision on the basis of section four of the Law on the Restoration of
the Professional Civil Service, I herewith forbid you, effective immediately, from
entering any government academic institution, and from using any State libraries
or scientific facilities.

Having followed his conscience, Dr. Krayer, like Else, had placed himself
and his family at risk, and had to leave Germany.

Peter's research with Dr. Krayer was formative and Janellen recalled that
Peter was a kind of "wunderkind" with science. He had never done research
before medical school but delved into fundamental science and received
a student award for research during medical school.

During this time Peter became interested in neuroscience. What is consciousness and pain? What is the brain's electrical activity during sleep or
lack of consciousness? It was during these years that Peter also developed an
interest in child neurology, a new field, focused on the care of children with
neurological diseases. In this he was heavily influenced by another of his
Harvard professors, Phil Dodge. Dodge was one of the first pediatric neurologists in the nation and started the first training program in child neurology at
Harvard. Peter committed to training in child neurology at both Massachusetts
General Hospital and Boston Children's Hospital.

A year after Peter started medical school, he and Janellen were married.
When asked to describe the Peter of those early years, Janellen recalled, "He
was tall and handsome. I soon learned he was this incredibly kind, fair fellow,
the kindest man on the planet." Peter and Janellen were married in June 1954
in a small outdoor ceremony at Max and Else's summer home in East Eden, NY,
among the rolling farm fields and woodlands of western New York State
(Figure 8.1). Else relished the opportunity to celebrate with her two sons
(Figure 8.2).

While Peter pursued his medical studies, Janellen pursued a PhD in psychology at Radcliffe College. At that time, Harvard College was all male.
Although the Radcliffe women had access to the same Harvard course work
and professors as did male students, Radcliffe College conferred degrees on
women. It was not until 1999 that Harvard and Radcliffe had fully merged and
all prior Radcliffe degrees were subsequently considered equivalent to
a Harvard University degree.

With limited financial resources, Peter and Janellen rented a run-down
apartment in Cambridge, MA, near the Harvard campus. These were formative years for both Peter and Janellen as they delved into understanding the
development of the human brain. They approached their questions from

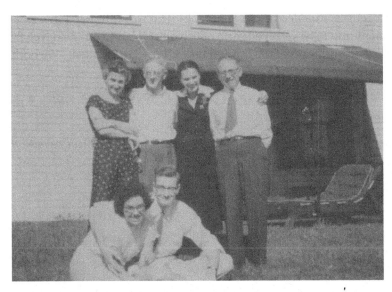

Figure 8.1 Peter and Janellen's wedding in East Eden, NY, at the home of Peter's parents. Left to right: Janellen's mother, Sylvia, Peter's stepfather Max, Else and Janellen's father Alan with the young couple.

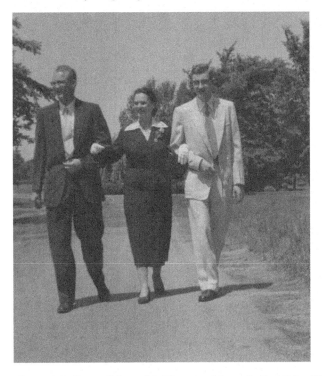

Figure 8.2 Else walking with Dieter and Peter in East Eden NY, after the wedding.

different perspectives, Janellen as a psychologist who was interested in cognitive development and Peter as a pediatric neurologist focused on the development and childhood diseases of the human brain. Janellen recalled: "We both enjoyed our work. How the brain works interested both of us."

References

1. A. Goldstein. Otto Krayer: October 22, 1899-March 18, 1982, *Biogr Mem Natl Acad Sci* 1987; **57**: 151–225.

9 UNDERSTANDING SLEEP AND CONSCIOUSNESS: RESEARCH AT THE NATIONAL INSTITUTES OF HEALTH

Following the Second World War, the United States experienced economic prosperity and, at the same time, turned away from its general policy of isolationism to one more focused on international engagement. The letter Peter wrote to his mother in 1948, before emigrating to the United States, was prescient. As noted in Chapter 6, Peter had written about his concerns over a *New York Times* article implying that America was already preparing and ready to enter another war, and had said, "I hope not." In 1949, the United States rejected its prior policy of having no military alliances in peacetime by forming the North Atlantic Treaty Organization (NATO) in response to the growing tensions between the United States and the Soviet Union. The first post-war US military engagement started shortly after Peter's US citizenship was confirmed. Else was relieved to have her sons in the US, but the concerns Richard and Else had written about were valid. Peter, as a US citizen, would be drafted into military service in the United States.

However, as a physician, Peter was eligible for the "Doctor Draft," which began at the outbreak of the Korean War and continued through the Vietnam War (1950–1973), allowing physicians to fulfill their military service obligations while doing medical research. The National Institutes of Health (NIH) was part of the Public Health Service and provided an alternative form of service for trained physicians. An option for fulfilling this commitment included performing research in the NIH Associate Training Program (ATP), the so-called "Yellow Berets." This break from clinical duties to focus on research allowed for physicians to train in science and bring a critical translational perspective of clinical relevance to basic biomedical research. The program was highly effective and succeeded in training many of the next generation of physician scientists and physician leaders [1]. Unlike current MD/PhD training programs in the United States that were developed in the 1980s, the NIH training occurred after completing medical school and/or part of residency training. Peter started in the NIH program in 1958 after completing his internship in internal medicine at Peter Bent Brigham and Women's Hospital in Boston, but before his clinical pediatric neurology training.

Peter was excited to embark upon basic neuroscience research. He had developed an interest in understanding how the electrical activity of the brain changed during sleep and wakefulness. For his research training, he selected the laboratory of a talented and energetic young physician scientist and psychiatrist, Ed Evarts, at the National Institutes of Mental Health (NIMH). Ed Evarts had been stationed on torpedo boats in the Navy during the Second World War but was subsequently taken out of the Navy to start his medical training at Harvard Medical School. He graduated from medical school in 1948 and then started an independent research program at the NIH using electrophysiology to understand changes in the activity of brain cells in the cortical regions of the brain under different conditions. Evarts had pioneered the methods to record the electrical activity (measured in voltage or current) in single cortical neurons in cats and monkeys. These recordings detect changes in electrical activity or electrical impulses that mediate communication between neurons. A large transient electrical signal, referred to as an action potential, travels along axons of the presynaptic neurons. This electrical activity triggers the release of a neurotransmitter at the synapse, where it affects the activity of the responding (post-synaptic) neuron, and can be detected by the electrophysiology methods that Evarts developed.

Evarts recruited several "Yellow Berets" into his research group, including Peter and a young psychiatrist, Irwin Feinberg, who later was the first person to propose that synaptic pruning is aberrant in schizophrenia. When interviewed in May 2022, Feinberg described the research environment in the Evarts laboratory as "terrific" and highly dynamic. Evarts was a meticulous scientist with a "fanatical attention to detail," but also with an openness to new ideas and the broad interests of his trainees. As Feinberg said, Evarts allowed them to do "whatever they wanted to do in the lab." Peter and Irwin did not work together on a project but were always friendly and supported each other. Feinberg said that Peter had "an instinct or judgement for what was important in a scientific problem – he showed that early on in Ed's lab. It was early years of sleep research, shortly after the discovery of REM sleep – and there were lots of nuggets to be picked up." He also recounted that "Peter first observed neural discharges during REM sleep, and his paper was incisive. Peter focused on a major issue and was not distracted – it was easy to get distracted in the early years of sleep research." Furthermore, Feinberg said: "Peter did an amazing study – it is still very important to sleep research – this work has deserved more attention than it has gotten."

Peter delved into laboratory research by recording the electrical activity of single cortical neurons in cats during both sleep and wakefulness. Before the 1950s, sleep was thought to be a passive state, like the brain's response to general anesthesia, where brain activity is dormant. However, in 1953, Aserinsky and Kleitman reported in a short letter to *Science* that eye movements increase in humans during sleep [2]. These authors elegantly recorded and quantified eye movements using an "electrooculogram" used to pick up eye movements during sleep. They found that detailed dreaming was associated with increased eye movements, or "ocular motility," later referred to as the REM phase of sleep.

Peter found something surprising in his recordings of single cortical neurons in sleeping cats. The "single unit activity" in some parts of the brain was higher during sleep than during waking. This study, published in *Science* in 1962, was the first to show that the electrical activity in the brain is higher during certain phases of sleep [3]. He found that during waking, there was more variance in the activity of individual neurons than during sleep. Neurons that fired rapidly during wakefulness tended to fire less rapidly during sleep. However, neurons with generally lower discharge rates tended to fire more during sleep than during waking. Altogether, Peter found that there was a generally higher neuronal discharge rate during sleep than during waking. The findings showed that there was a general change in the pattern of electrical activity in the brain during sleep, and that sleep did not represent a quiescent phase of the brain's electrical activity. Sleep is an active electrical state. In contrast to the unresponsive state of a patient under anesthesia, like the "Ether Dome" patient (with relatively constant brain waves), they found that sleep is entirely different, with cycles of more and less brain activity.

As Peter's long-time friend and Nobel Prize winner Eric Kandel said in a message for Peter's memorial service, in September 2013, "What is less often considered is Peter was outstanding from the very beginning of his career." Eric continued:

His first two articles were extraordinary. In his work with Ed Evarts at NIH, he was one of the first people to record electrical activity in the brain from living animals. He recorded from the visual system of animals. He discovered that the firing patterns changed with different periods of sleep and wakefulness. And this was one of the first precursors to the insight that sleep is not uniform – that there are periods of greater activity and periods of less activity. And as it later turned out, periods of greater activity are associated with REM sleep, with dreaming sleep. Peter was one of the precursors of appreciating the different phases of sleep. This was a fabulous contribution.

Making an important finding can be transformative for a junior scientist, and Peter's findings with Ed Evarts changed thinking about brain dormancy and sleep. However, as was often the case with Peter, as Feinberg said, "he was humble and quiet about his accomplishments." He did not bring attention to his work and he was not comfortable being the "salesman." Feinberg recalled that Peter was sometimes "unbending – he was a hard man in some respects" and did not "suffer fools gladly." Also, "Peter had a harsh opinion of people getting a lot of attention in science – the showy people in science." Feinberg said that Peter shared this disdain with Ed Evarts and, together, the three of them would make fun of the big shots at NIH – people who spoke eloquently but did not have much substance with their science. This hesitancy on the part of Peter for showmanship surely hindered his science, especially later in his career. He struggled at times with NIH funding and hesitated to advertise his discovery of synaptic pruning. Indeed, it was not until the early 2000s when someone else told me that my father had discovered synaptic pruning that I realized the magnitude of his work. It is certainly possible that, if he had had more of a flare for promotion, others would have grasped the importance of synaptic pruning earlier and it would have expedited further discovery in the field. He might have run a large laboratory group and followed up his findings in more diverse ways. It is also possible that acceptance of his new findings simply required time, and corroboration by other scientists. But what was clear early on is that Peter knew how to go after the important questions in science. Feinberg said, "Peter did not waste his time on trivial projects just to get papers published – other people did this to beef up their CVs. Peter quietly focused and discerned and knew how to choose a problem worth working on – Peter was a genius at that." During the years in the Evarts laboratory, Peter's thinking about science was transformed. Even after years of clinical work that distracted Peter from science, Peter continued in the ways of his mentor Ed Evarts, and throughout his career approached science with a similar "fanatical attention to detail."

In addition to the science, Peter and Janellen enjoyed an active social life with the neuroscience community at NIH. Feinberg recalled that "Janellen was wonderful – brilliant and charming. She had a great relationship with Peter and he respected her, and he respected her independence." Janellen was the more outgoing of the pair – and formed close friendships with some of the career-oriented wives of the "Yellow Berets." Ed Evarts' wife, Josephine, was a colorful scientist from the south, who was unconventional and outspoken. Janellen, who went on to become an internationally recognized cognitive psychologist, formed a close and lifelong friendship with Denise Kandel, a social scientist and wife of Eric Kandel. Both Janellen and Denise were completing their PhDs remotely as their husbands worked at NIH. As Feinberg said about Eric Kandel, "Eric was ambitious, more ambitious than I realized then, but very congenial. At the time he was a clinically oriented neuroscientist – charming and a jokester." And as Irwin happily understated, "it all turned out very well for him." Eric Kandel, together with Arvid Carlsson and Paul Greengard, won the Nobel Prize in Physiology or Medicine for his discoveries related to memory and signal transduction in the nervous system of a simple model organism, the sea slug *Aplysia*.

Like Peter, both Eric and Denise Kandel were immigrants from Europe, and they formed an immediate connection that – together with their interests in neuroscience, music and art – led to a close friendship as they raised their families together in Washington, DC, then Boston, and then the New York area (Figure 9.1). They also developed a shared interest in expressionist art and explored remote art galleries in the search of new art. Each family still owns copies of the same Max Beckman print, of a lady with an askance gaze and a pearl necklace. German expressionist art reflected the angst in Germany

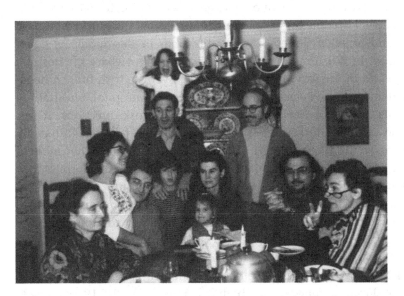

Figure 9.1 Photo from one of the holiday gatherings with family friends. From left, Denise Kandel, Janellen, Peter and Eric Kandel with children. Next, neuroscientist Alden Spencer and family, and Joel Spiegelman with his wife Gail.

before and during the war and stimulated an obsessive interest of Peter's throughout his life – the raw human emotion and hidden angst that he rarely spoke about. Although each of their stories were different, Peter, Eric and Denise all shared this angst having grown up in Europe during the war. Unlike Peter, both Eric and Denise came from Jewish families. Eric was born in Vienna and fled the country when he was nine with his older brother, to join his uncle in New York City where they were later joined by his parents. But Denise, like Peter, spent all of her childhood in Europe during the war. Denise was raised in a secular Jewish family in France before the war and was placed in a convent for safety during the war. The nuns of Sainte-Jeanne d'Arc of Cahors safeguarded Denise and raised her as a Catholic. Denise later said (February 14, 2022) that she knew "more about Catholicism than the Jewish faith," and even took her first communion in the convent. Denise's father survived his years in an internment camp south of Paris and Denise reunited with her family after the war, then immigrated to the United States in 1949, arriving there around the time that Peter did. During these years Peter rarely spoke about his childhood experiences in Germany, to his friends or even to Janellen. As a *Kriegskind* (war child), Peter responded as a classic post-Second World War stoic. His friends Denise and Eric were more forthcoming about their pasts. Peter worked to forget, or at least to not tell. It was not until many years later that he began to share stories from his childhood.

During the NIH years, Peter and Janellen welcomed their first child. The story of his arrival became an oft-told tale that reflected the quirky humor of both Peter and Janellen. Janellen went into labor in the middle of a hot summer's night in Washington, DC. Peter did not know where the hospital was but drove forth anyway, in their dilapidated vehicle with broken head-lights. Janellen described Peter nervously driving to the hospital, uncertain of where he was going but unwilling to pull over and ask directions. It was difficult to navigate the darker streets without headlights. Janellen, grimacing in labor, shined a flashlight out of the front window of the car as they maneu-vered their way. As they approached what they thought was the hospital they were greeted by "large guards with massive machine guns," who promptly turned them away. They had arrived at the Pentagon! Flustered and confused, and suppressing his lifelong disdain of authority, Peter turned around, unsure of where to go. They were pleasantly surprised when a nearby police officer took pity on the young couple and escorted them to the hospital. Their joint retelling of the story was classic Peter and Janellen: cheerful deprecation, enjoyment of slapstick comedy. They both loved the weekly US 1960s comedy show *Rowan and Martin's Laugh-In* and the family rarely missed an episode. Peter would laugh uproariously during the hour-long shows riddled with "ridiculous" political and social commentary. *Laugh-In* was the source of a punch-line they injected at the end of stories for rest of their lives, whether discussing people or science: "And that's the truth."

References

1. S. Khot, B. S. Park and W.T. Longstreth. The Vietnam War and medical research: Untold legacy of the US Doctor Draft and the NIH "Yellow Berets." *Acad Med* 2011; **86**: 502–8.
2. E. Aserinsky and N. Kleitman. Regularly occurring periods of eye motility, and concomitant phenomena. *Science* 1953; **118**: 273–4.
3. E. V. Evarts, T. C. Fleming and P. R. Huttenlocher. Recovery cycle of visual cortex of the awake and sleeping cat. *Science* 1962; **135**: 736–8.

10 ENTERING THE COGNITIVE REVOLUTION: NEUROSCIENCE AND COGNITIVE PSYCHOLOGY

The Cognitive Revolution was an intellectual movement in the 1950s and 1960s focused on using the scientific method to understand human cognition, otherwise known as the process of learning and memory. This revolution in the field of psychology was happening at the same time that neuroscientists like Hubel and Wiesel were exploring how neurons in the brain are organized to enable behaviors such as visual perception. It was in this environment that both Peter and Janellen developed further as scientists. The connections between their respective fields provided fodder for discussion and debate throughout their careers. Peter focused on cellular events and biological processes in developmental neuroscience, while Janellen probed the mechanisms of human verbal and mathematical learning and memory.

Returning to Boston after a few whirlwind years at the National Institutes of Health was a shocking transition for both Peter and Janellen. Peter had to jump back into the demanding hours of clinical training in neurology at Massachusetts General Hospital (MGH), often clocking 100 hours per week in the hospital (Figure 10.1). During these years Peter spent more time with his neurology colleagues at MGH than with his own family (Figure 10.2). Peter's mother Else commented more than once: "Janellen, you really are as good as an heiress," referring to Janellen providing both the care for their growing family and the financial support while Peter engaged in clinical training with limited pay. In the 1950s and 1960s, the era of the "happy homemaker," Janellen worked full-time jobs. She finished her PhD and started a postdoctoral fellowship at Harvard in the Department of Psychology. In the midst of the Cognitive Revolution, Janellen was well prepared for the quantitative focus of this new field because she had completed her PhD with a talented statistician, Professor

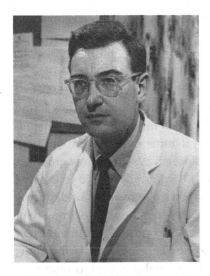

Figure 10.1 Peter Huttenlocher as a young doctor.

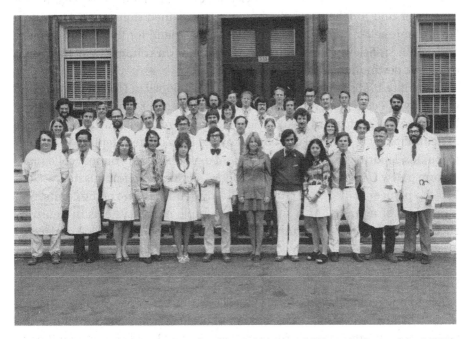

Figure 10.2 Photo of the Neurology faculty, residents and fellows in front of the MGH in the early 1960s.

Frederick Mosteller. On the scientific publication database PubMed Janellen's first listed publication is a single-authored paper entitled "Development of formal reasoning on concept formation problems," published in *Child Development* in 1964.

Peter and Janellen searched for a place to live in Boston close to the MGH, so that Peter could see his family during breaks in his work schedule. They found a dilapidated old brownstone home on Myrtle Street in the Beacon Hill neighborhood of Boston. They could not afford to buy a home, even in what was then a run-down neighborhood, but a close friend of Janellen's and fellow graduate student from Radcliffe, the economist Barbara Bergmann, offered to pay the down payment on the home. They swiftly formed an agreement and, during the next years, between shifts in the hospital, Peter spent his spare time – with his children close by – fixing up this old home. The house is in the now very upscale and gentrified Beacon Hill neighborhood. Ironically, at the time, break-ins and other disruptions were common. One dark night, a man who was climbing over a wall in the rear of their home was met by Peter holding the nearest thing he could grab – an alarm clock – out of the window and shouting – in his thick German accent – "Get out or I will shoot!" It worked. By the time Peter and Janellen sold the home it had gained significantly in value. Peter and Janellen were able to pay back their friend for the down payment and retain sufficient funds for a down payment on a home near their next academic destination, Yale University.

In the late 1950s, a neuroscience hub was developed at Harvard University. Otto Krayer, Peter's first research mentor and the chair of the Department of Pharmacology at Harvard Medical School, recognized the growing importance of neurobiology to the field of pharmacology. He recruited Stephen W. Kuffler to join his department, and Kuffler brought a group of four younger colleagues to form a new Department of Neurobiology. Kuffler was a famous neuroscientist who pioneered the use of crayfish to study dendrites, one of the connecting projections of neurons. As a supporter of simple model systems in neuroscience, Kuffler provided important support and mentorship for Eric Kandel and his work with the sea slug *Aplysia*. The core faculty recruited by Kuffler included significant young talent: David Hubel, Torsten Wiesel, Ed Furshpan and David Potter.

Key to navigating these years for Janellen was her network of career-oriented women friends, whose success as females in academia was not common in the late 1950s and early 1960s. During Janellen's PhD and postdoctoral training she developed a close and lifelong friendship with David Potter's wife, Molly Potter, a fellow PhD student and postdoctoral fellow at Harvard in cognitive psychology. Molly Potter, Denise Kandel and the economist Barbara Bergmann were all close friends of Janellen who combined successful academic careers with raising children, which was even more unusual at that time. Indeed, Janellen, Molly and Denise were all pregnant at the same time in 1961. Peter and Janellen socialized frequently with this network of neuroscientists and psychologists, many of whom went on to remarkable scientific careers. Molly Potter became a named professor at Massachusetts Institute of Technology, with interests in rapid visual processing. She discovered that people understand pictures faster than writing. Denise Kandel became a professor at Columbia University and studied the sequence of first-time use of various legal and illegal drugs. Barbara Bergmann worked for multiple US government agencies, University of Maryland and American University, as a feminist economist focused on increasing the status of women. There is no question that this network of female and male colleagues/friends/spouses provided an important influence for both Janellen and Peter. They provided uncommon examples of how both women and men could successfully balance high-powered careers with long-term marriages and child rearing.

Peter was the only member of this group who continued with clinical medicine and basic science. Eric Kandel had initially pursued dual clinical (psychoanalysis) and basic research in his first faculty position at Harvard Medical School. As quoted in Eric's book *In Search of Memory*, his wife Denise said to him at the time: "What, compromise your scientific career by trying to combine basic research with clinical practice and administrative responsibilities!" [1]. Eric agreed that his basic research goals were not compatible with continued clinical work, and in the mid-1960s the Kandels moved to New York City where Eric built his very successful scientific career.

Peter made a different decision and did both clinical medicine and science for the rest of his career. Carter Snead, his first fellow at Yale, later said: "Peter taught me to be a clinician and a scientist before there was such a term." After completing clinical training, Peter performed fundamental research as a junior faculty member at Harvard Medical School. During this time Peter published a Letter (peer-reviewed paper) in *Nature*, in 1966, entitled "Development of neuronal activity in the neocortex of the kitten" [2]. In that paper he wrote: "The results indicate that large parts of neocortex in the kitten are electrically silent at birth, but that neuronal activity rapidly develops in the postnatal period." This was one of his first studies trying to address the developmental changes in brain connections, in this case using single neuron recordings. He concluded: "The earliest activity in cortical neurons shows little of the complexity seen in the adult cerebral cortex." This question – how the brain normally develops and makes connections over development – drove his future research on synaptogenesis during human brain development.

The Nobel Prize-winning work of David Hubel and Torsten Wiesel on the plasticity of neuronal connections in the visual system (described in Chapter 2) had a significant influence on Peter. Their discovery that there is a window of plasticity during the development of the visual system provided important new insights into the mammalian brain. Understanding this plasticity became a major focus of the later work of both Peter and Janellen, who asked: How does the environment influence brain development and childhood learning?

References

1. E. R Kandel. *In Search of Memory: The Emergence of a New Science of the Mind.* W. W. Norton & Company, 2006.
2. P. R. Huttenlocher. Development of neuronal activity in neocortex of the kitten. *Nature* 1966; **211**: 91–2.

11 PHYSICIAN FIRST, SCIENTIST SECOND?

Case history of a killer disease: Reye's syndrome: a medical mystery

This year in the wake of an outbreak of influenza B virus 250 cases of Reye's syndrome have been reported in the United States, with 90 deaths ...

1970s newspaper headline and article opening in *Ann Arbor News*

Peter arrived as a new assistant professor of pediatric neurology at Yale University in 1966. This was in the midst of the Reye's syndrome peak of the late 1960s. Reye's syndrome is a life-threatening pediatric disease characterized by progressive brain and liver damage in children, often after a viral illness. It became a rare condition after epidemiological studies suggested a link between aspirin use in children and the onset of Reye's syndrome after a viral illness. The reduced rates of Reye's syndrome are largely attributable to public health messaging to limit aspirin use in children, but until that change, it often fell to pediatric neurologists to keep Reye's syndrome patients alive.

Based on clinical demand, Peter allowed clinical pediatric neurology to consume the largest share of his professional time and attention (Figure 11.1). One of Peter's medical colleagues, Gabe Mirkin, noted in his online newsletter (DrMirkin.com) in September 2013: "In 1962, when I was a resident at the Massachusetts General Hospital, Peter often consulted on my neurology patients. He would write 30 page-long hand-written histories and physicals on my patients, the result of hour-long interviews (other consultants rarely wrote more than a couple pages or spent more than a few minutes with the patients)." One can ponder whether modern care-tracking medical systems would now tolerate such clinical inefficiency. Peter showed similar commitment to patients with Reye's syndrome. In the 1960s and 1970s the treatment of these patients could be all-consuming. As neurologist Carter Snead put it, during an interview in May 2022, "The kids died left and right." Peter would guide their treatment directly in the intensive care unit at all hours of the day and night. Inevitably, this left Peter with less time and less mental space for his scientific research. However,

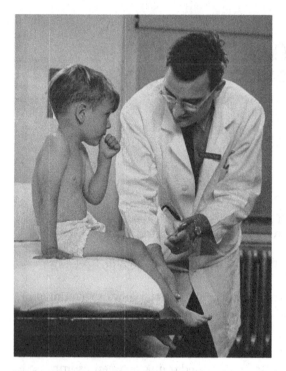

Figure 11.1 Peter with a patient, performing a patellar reflex test.

he became a spokesperson for the care and management of patients with Reye's syndrome and developed a national reputation in the area (Figure 11.2).

The scientist portions of Peter's activities, while given less time, were never fully set aside. Carter Snead was Peter's first clinical fellow as a faculty member at Yale University. He later became head of the Department of Neurology at the Hospital for Sick Children at University of Toronto, and a lead researcher in the basic science of epilepsy. Snead remembered that Peter:

> had an unbelievable wide range of intellect. An amazing clinician – watching him do an exam provided a wonderful synthesis of clinical findings. He was a true physician scientist before it was even a term . . . He taught me to do research – I did not even know which end of a test tube was up . . . He knew I was interested in epilepsy – and suggested an experiment. The experiment worked and launched my entire research career on the basic science of epilepsy.

Snead was only warming up, as he went on to say: "[Peter] did ground breaking work that opened new fields – and then let someone else fill in the details." He was "visionary." He was a "Golly gee whiz kind of guy – nothing

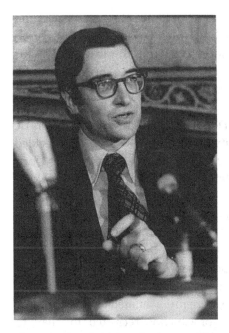

Figure 11.2 Yale University image of Peter talking to the media about Reye's syndrome in New Haven, Connecticut, in the early 1970s.

fake about it – this is how he was – wide eyed with curiosity about everything – and this masked an unbelievable intellect."

One of the highest-impact outcomes from Peter's time at Yale was that he pioneered the ketogenic diet for epilepsy. He devised a very - low - carbohydrate, high - saturated - fat diet that was palatable and showed that it worked for epilepsy. Snead noted, "it is still a second-line therapy for the treatment of children with epilepsy." A ketogenic diet was first tried in the 1920s, but it never caught on because the children refused to eat it. Peter showed that medium-chain triglyceride (MCT) oil worked and made it palatable. He made an "MCT ice cream" and also went on to show it was effective. Published in *Pediatric Research* in 1976, he reported improved epilepsy control in children with intractable seizures [1]. The "MCT" diet, comprised of 60% MCT oil and a more palatable combination of protein and carbohydrates, replaced the classic ketogenic diet for use in children with epilepsy.

Snead said that Peter told him, "If you are a clinician scientist – when you are in the lab putzing around – PhD colleagues think you are a dabbler since you are not there full - time." He went on to say that clinician scientists have a "huge disadvantage in the grant game. However, the advantages are huge – you can see clinical ramifications – Peter taught me this. He had the vision and saw the importance of synaptogenesis – and what it meant for the developing brain – he used to talk to me about it" (this was well before Peter's discoveries about synaptic pruning). As Eric Kandel later said about this discovery, in his message for Peter's memorial service, "He saw implications of his findings that many people who had only had a basic science background might have overlooked."

It was for all of these reasons that Doris Trauner, currently a pediatric neurologist and professor at the University of California – San Diego, decided to do her pediatric neurology training with Peter at Yale. Shortly after Doris signed on to train at Yale, Peter called to let her know that he would be looking for a job in Chicago. She was stunned that this "famous" talented pediatric neurologist was following his wife to Chicago and had yet to find a job. The move was triggered because Janellen, a rising talent on the Teachers College (Graduate School of Education) faculty at Columbia University, was unable to procure a job at the Yale University Department of Psychology. As Janellen said: "they were explicitly not interested in hiring female faculty" at the time. Professor positions at research universities were rarely offered to women in the 1960s and 1970s. When the University of Chicago recruited Janellen to a prestigious chaired professorship, Peter and Janellen decided it was time to make a move. a move was also motivated by the long commutes to New Haven and New York, which were taxing for a family that now included three children.

Peter started a faculty position at the University of Chicago School of Medicine in 1974. Doris Trauner decided to make the move to the University of Chicago with Peter. She said that, at the time, few people were interested in taking female trainees and he was very supportive. Trauner already had a publication in the Reye's syndrome field, and he supported her independent pursuit of this project during her training. In an interview in February 2022, she said: "I had the freedom to do what I wanted" and was assisted by Peter's technician Fran at the University of Chicago. While Trauner worked on Reye's syndrome she watched with wonder as Peter spent hours at the electron microscope, imaging synapses. He did not have a team. He did this work alone and let Trauner pursue her independent interests. She said: "It was amazing; he did it himself, and his work is still quoted all of the time in pediatric neurology and developmental neuroscience." Peter was a "thought leader" in human developmental neuroscience.

Doris Trauner recalled sitting for hours in Peter's office stacked high with journals and papers in seeming chaos, discussing patients and science. Hours of one-on-one mentoring. He enjoyed what he did and was enthusiastic about both the clinic and research. He was a *creative thinker – he would talk about something outside of his field and he would have creative ideas – he was fun to talk to – a superb clinician and diagnostician . . . you do not come across people like that often. He instilled this into the people he trained – you spend time thinking about what is going on with the patient – what is causing this? Do not take anything for granted. He was thorough and precise, and modeled critical thinking.*

Trauner did, however, note that Peter was not a very good administrator. He was "kind and modest and never wanted to do anything to get recognition – he did it because he thought it was the right thing to do." However, if someone was hired and failed to do a good job, he did not deal with the problem. He avoided conflict and did not handle administration – above or below him – well. He never fired anyone. As Snead said, "Peter had a kind of naivete and inno-cence" – and was not good for administration "because he was too trusting of everyone."

The Child Neurology Residency Training Program at the University of Chicago was begun in 1976 by Peter. The program has trained a cohort of pediatric neurology fellows who are now professors at universities across the United States. The former fellows gather yearly at the pediatric neurology meetings to dine – in years past with Peter present – and they still continue this tradition in his absence. When Peter started at the University of Chicago, neurology was in chaos. Adult neurology had been decimated and the entire team had relocated to another university. Pediatric neurology was under the control of the chair of the Department of Pediatrics, who seemingly did not have interest in neurology and was not supportive of the pediatric neurology program, financially or otherwise. Peter was a kind of "spousal hire" and had limited negotiating power (or skill) to advocate for the team. After Peter's arrival, Barry Arnason became the new director of adult neurology, and recruited a team of neurologists that enlivened the adult team and interfaced well with pediatric neurology (Figure 11.3). However, they did not have the power to make the work conditions better for Peter in the Department of Pediatrics.

Peter also started a learning disabilities clinic at the University of Chicago. This clinic was the first of its kind in the nation. In clinic, Peter worked with faculty member Susan Levine, a developmental psychologist who also worked with Janellen. Levine said, in an interview in February 2022: "the kids loved him. . . . He saw complicated patients with difficult diseases and the families were struggling. Peter gave them hope – not false hope – but he believed in the plasticity of the brain and the capacity for the children to improve. He also gave the families strategies to cope and how to work with their child."

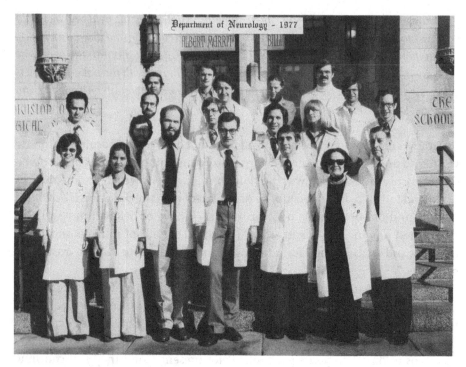

Figure 11.3 University of Chicago Neurology faculty, including Peter's first pediatric neurology fellow at the University of Chicago, Doris Trauner.

Peter also enjoyed training medical students. He was a popular medical school professor, both in the lecture hall and at the patient's bedside. A former medical student and joint recipient of the 2011 Nobel Prize in Physiology or Medicine, Bruce Beutler, was quoted in the University of Chicago magazine as recalling that Peter Huttenlocher's mode of instruction was "teaching by example." "From him I first learned that children, and in particular infants are almost like a different species. They must be examined for neurological function using entirely different tests and evaluation criteria than adults." Beutler also noted that Reye's syndrome was alarmingly common in those years: "I remember such a patient, a boy who was treated with aspirin when he had chicken pox and had a severe encephalopathy. Peter seemed deeply moved . . . I remember him calling out to the comatose child by name, hoping for a response."

After Peter's passing, one of his former Reye's syndrome patients, now a tenured professor, emailed me with the subject: Thanks to your dad for saving my life.

Dear Anna,

Pardon me for contacting you unsolicited and out of the blue, but my mother sent me Peter Huttenlocher's obituary, and through some googling, I found that you're his daughter and you're at UW–Madison [University of Wisconsin–Madison], which is where I got my PhD, and your father saved my life, so the confluence of all those facts made me really want to reach out to you. The life-saving part involves me at age 8 contracting Reye's syndrome following my receiving aspirin for a fever. I have almost no recollection of the events, but my parents told me that after getting chicken pox, I started acting weird. My pediatrician didn't think much of it and sent me home with a pat on the head, but my grandma was visiting us then, and I apparently hit her and told her I hated her, and from this she recognized instantly that I was not right. So my parents brought me back to the doctor, and I subsequently ended up under the treatment of your father. While in the hospital, I slipped into a coma for two days, and my mom tells me your father stayed at the hospital for the whole time. She said when I finally emerged from the coma, he reacted like "a proud papa." Again, I don't remember any of this, but I can now obviously recognize what this meant, and my mom sent me a long letter detailing the whole experience after seeing your father's obituary. Long part of the story short, after being saved by your father, I got through middle & high school, went to college at University of Illinois, then went to grad school at UW-Madison, where I got my PhD in film studies. I then got a job teaching film studies, published a book, got tenure, got married, and all along have had an extremely happy life. So … it feels weird to email someone to say, "Thanks to your dad for saving my life!" but I did want to share this thought nonetheless. Though I don't remember much of what I went through, your dad's name and his dogged pursuit of medical knowledge will forever mean the world to me and my family. I am so sorry for your loss (and humanity's loss), but I hope that hearing of his impact on one life will serve some value.

Thanks, and bless you and your family

In another former-patient encounter, this time unrelated to Reye's syndrome, I was approached after teaching Immunology to undergraduates at the UW–Madison. A student, Andrew, came up to me after class and said: "Your father was my doctor." Andrew's mother subsequently described his condition in an email:

It was late summer in 1995, when we went to our family doctor and he had no idea what was wrong with Andrew. He told us to make an appointment with

Dr. Huttenlocher because he said if anyone can make a diagnosis it would be him. At the appointment, Dr. Huttenlocher asked about Andrew's symptoms. I was surprised that he did not physically examine Andrew, but he asked him to go to the long hallway outside his office and walk back and forth. As Andrew was walking back towards us, Dr. Huttenlocher said that Andrew has strep and needs to be tested, that he has rheumatic chorea that would get better in about 8 weeks and that he needed to see a pediatric cardiologist for any possible heart damage. I was amazed that he could tell all this by Andrew just walking in the hallway. What struck me was his calm demeanor and his assurance that this was all manageable. It was a relief. He also told us that there used to be hospital wards with children with rheumatic chorea and that he had not seen any case in about 20 years. We are looking forward to reading the book when it is published and sharing it with our family.

Andrew said:

When I was a child of ~10 years I remember having a very bad cold/flu and feeling the worst I had ever felt, I also had hives all over, and later a type of palsy on one side of my body. My pediatrician was flummoxed, and referred me to a specialist and children's hospital by the University of Chicago, Dr. Huttenlocher. I remember he was a kind older man with a European accent who reminded me of my Grandpa. He quickly diagnosed me with rheumatic chorea, and referred me to a pediatric cardiologist as my heart may have been damaged. I then was put on a prophylaxis treatment of penicillin to prevent me from getting strep throat again and causing another reaction. I had some heart damage due to my illness that if Dr. Huttenlocher had not treated early enough I may have died or had permanent heart problems. Thankfully, my heart healed during my teenage years, and I no longer have a heart murmur. I remember how Dr. Huttenlocher had a great bedside manner as he addressed me, a precocious child at the time, with respect, like an adult.

Peter habitually talked to children like they were adults. Trauner also noted "he treated everyone equally" – women, men, his patients – "he treated everyone with the same amount of respect and consideration – patients from all backgrounds." The boy from Germany may have found his greatest calling as a physician, taking care of patients.

References

1. P. R. Huttenlocher. Ketonemia and seizures: Metabolic and anticonvulsant effects of two ketogenic diets in childhood epilepsy. *Pediatr Res* 1976; **10**: 536–40.

12 COMPARATIVE BRAIN REGIONS AND SYNAPSE FORMATION

Good science has a kind of rebellion nature to it – antiauthor-
itarian and mischievous – without this bit of fun many of us
would not be doing science
Itai Yinai PhD, New York University (on Twitter, 2022)

Peter was always thinking about synapses – even early on with
the sleep studies.
Janellen Huttenlocher

As his former National Institutes of Health (NIH) colleague Irwin Feinberg put
it, Peter's research "took a 180-degree turn" after his move to the University of
Chicago in 1974. Instead of focusing on the brains of patients with neurological deficits, he started to study the "gridwork" of healthy brains. As Peter
said, "the findings in the normal population were more interesting than the
abnormal population." His landmark 1979 study published in *Brain Research*
was unexpected [1]. The accepted thinking at that time was that brains actually get more connections as we learn and develop, but he found the opposite
to be true. After a burst of new synapses form in the first year of life, unneeded
connections are removed, or pruned. All scientific discoveries are incremental
and build on the work of other scientists. But rarely, a scientific discovery can
also present an entirely new way of thinking about a problem – and is truly
a breakthrough. In a conversation in May 2022, Feinberg said about Peter's
work: "the idea of brain connections was not in the thinking in the 1980s. The
skeptics were many."

In 1993, a *Chicago Tribune* reporter, Ronald Kotulak, interviewed Peter for an
article entitled "Mental workouts pump up brain power." Kotulak wrote:

*As he focused on one sample and then another, Huttenlocher was astonished by
the sharply increasing number of brain-cell connections; he later compared the site
to watching the slow-motion frames of an explosion. A sample from a 28-week-old*

fetus totaled 124 million connections between cells; the sample from a newborn, 253 million; and the sample from an 8-month-old infant – an amazing 572 million connections, findings that defied conventional scientific wisdom. "It was a strange thing to see," he said. "The number of connections kept going up and up and up and then they started to go down." Brain connections, he soon learned, start to fizzle toward the end of the first year of life, stabilizing at 354 million per speck of brain tissue by age 12.

Habitually self-effacing, Peter's next comment was "I stumbled on the whole thing. It was something that nobody expected. It took quite a long time until people began to accept that this really happens."

Kotulak followed this up with journalistic flair:

By the time he was done with his census, Huttenlocher not only stunned neuroscientists with his demonstration of how fast the brain initially develops, he also provided a glimpse of the brain's raw power to create a powerful learning machine .... . Huttenlocher's pioneering census was the first hint of something that has evolved into accepted scientific fact today: the brain is not a static organ; it is a constantly changing mass of cell connections that are deeply affected by experience and hold the key to human intelligence.

The 1993 *Chicago Tribune* article was written 14 years after the publication of Peter's 1979 paper in *Brain Research*. Rather than "stunning" neuroscientists, the response of much of the neuroscience community to the 1979 publication was more one of disinterest or skepticism. As Chris Walsh said in conversation in December 2021, at the time "some people thought it was a folly, although it ended up being robust and durable science." Walsh noted that there was skepticism because the electron microscope was used to study only a "small grid of brain tissue, and the sample size was small." People were "put off by the scale of it." How do you say something informative about human brain development through the lens of a small speck of tissue? It was difficult to grapple with. Feinberg's comment about the response to the discovery of synapse elimination was: "Science is truth by consensus. It takes time."

Despite his own skepticism, when Peter first noticed the dramatic changes in synapse number in normal human brains, he knew it was important. He knew the work had to be done with "fanatical" attention to detail. In the methods section of his 1979 paper [1], Peter concisely described his handling of the brain tissue. The careful work of laboratory science was described in language that some readers will view with trepidation and others, like Peter, will genuinely enjoy:

> *Middle frontal gyrus was chosen for study, since considerable developmental data on this region of cortex in the human are available, especially as regards development of dendritic branching in cortical neurons. Cases with known neurologic disease or with severe prolonged hypoxia prior to death were excluded. Small blocks of cortex, including layers 1–3, were removed at autopsy and were fixed in 5% glutaraldehyde in phosphate buffer (0.3 M, pH 7.4). The tissue was prepared for electron microscopy by the phosphotungstic acid method of Bloom and Aghajanian, which stains synaptic profiles selectively. Thin sections (silver interference color, about 75 nm in thickness) were cut with a Sorvall MT2 microtome, and were examined in an RCA Elmoscope 4 electron microscope. Photographs were taken of layer 3 frontal cortex in a random fashion at magnification of 6800. Finished prints were 2.5 times magnifications of the negatives, for a total magnification of 17,000. Twenty to thirty 8 Å ~10 inch prints were prepared for each sample, and identifiable synaptic profiles were enumerated in each print. Only profiles with clearly identifiable presynaptic projections, synaptic cleft and dense postsynaptic band were counted. Mean synapse count per cu.mm [cubic millimetre] was calculated for each sample.*

Although surprising, there was a context for these findings. Changeux and Danchin, in an opinion piece published in *Nature* in 1976, proposed that biochemical signals alone were not sufficient to explain the complexity of neuronal connections during development [2]. They postulated that an increase in specificity of the connections is derived from the stabilization of particular synapses and the regression of others. The authors provide a biochemical perspective for Peter's finding that there is an explosive change in synapses in the developing human brain. It also set the stage for Changeux's later hypothesis that early synaptic connections are random, with the persistence of the used synapses and the regression of the unused connections.

After the publication of his 1979 study and the tepid response from the neuroscience community, Peter knew more work had to be done. Was the burst in synapses in early childhood and their subsequent elimination happening in other regions of the brain? Was the timing similar to what he observed in the frontal gyrus? To do this research he needed more tissue and there were significant challenges to performing post-mortem brain studies, which continue to this day. It was difficult to get samples in the

United States, and for synapse quantification the samples needed to include unfixed brain tissue. Samples were difficult or close to impossible to obtain in the United States because few autopsies were done on children or young adults who died suddenly with no apparent illness. It was around this time that Peter attended a meeting of the Society of Neuroscience, the international conference that gathers neuroscientists from around the world to present their work every year. Peter was interested in working with Hendrik Van der Loos, a neurobiologist in Lausanne. Van der Loos, a developmental neurobiologist, had recently published the first electron microscopy (EM) study to examine synapse number and density in the human cerebral cortex from the neonatal period [3]. The EM method was a much more accurate way to quantify synapse density than the traditional Golgi method. Van der Loos and colleagues showed that synapse formation started in the second trimester during neonatal development, prior to the completion of the developmental neuronal migration that occurs in the fetal brain. Peter used a similar approach to study synaptogenesis but modified it to quantify synapse number in the brain during development using the phosphotungstic acid method that selectively stained peri-synaptic proteins, making it easier to quantify synapse density.

At the Society of Neuroscience meeting shortly after the publication of his 1979 study Peter met with Van der Loos, who at that time directed the Institute of Anatomy at the University of Lausanne in Switzerland. Hendrik was an expert on the development of synapses in the neonatal cortex of mice, and immediately grasped the importance of Peter's findings on synaptic elimination in the human brain. He was eager to help. Hendrik had access to brain samples from the autopsies of healthy children and adults, since it was common practice to perform autopsies even on healthy people who died in accidents in Switzerland. At the meeting, Peter and Hendrik forged a plan. In collaboration with Van der Loos, Peter looked at synapses during development in the human visual cortex (striate cortex). He acquired critical samples that would later allow the analysis of patterns of synaptogenesis in other regions of the brain.

Peter lived in Lausanne, Switzerland, in the summer and fall of 1982 and returned to work with Hendrik in subsequent summers. During a sabbatical in 1982, Peter and Janellen lived in the small village of Lutry in the vineyards, five kilometers from Lausanne. There was a network of trails through the vineyards near their apartment in Lutry, on the hilly slopes above Lake Geneva. The vineyards were reminiscent of the trails in the vineyards surrounding his grandparent's home near Stuttgart. During that summer he sent me the following in a letter:

> *We had a very good visit to Venezia. That is, the drive there was very long, monotonous and hot. But Venice was as unusual and beautiful as last time. Carl liked it too – especially feeding bread to the hundreds of pigeons in St. Marks square and stroking the many Venetian cats. He also became quite independent and took long strolls alone. They had a large Picasso visit in Venice – quite interesting. He was certainly his best as a young man from about 1900 to 1920. But then in very old age until his death in 1971, he did some pretty good work again. On the way back we took a different route – much more interesting. Along Lago Magione and then the Simphon pass (between 6–7,000 feet high). There still was some snow at the highest point and we walked around and threw snowballs in June! We had some bad news from the states. My research grant application for NIH was "approved but not funded." This means I will no longer have money for research, and I am quite depressed about it. That is about all of the news from Lausanne. I still love the beauty and quiet of this place. This weekend we take off again for Paris.*

For many years, Peter struggled to fund his synaptogenesis work. Was this because it was ahead of its time? Was it viewed as "folly" to do these types of studies using the human brain? Or was this a gap with Peter's skill as a research group leader? Is it because he struggled to sell his work and tell his story in a way that convinced other neuroscientists? There has long been criticism that NIH funds safe science and has less inclination for out-of-the-box thinking. Descriptive science is particularly difficult to fund, yet Peter needed the funding to do his work as time on the electron microscope was expensive. Whenever possible, Peter worked with Hendrik in Lausanne but the gap in NIH funding significantly hindered his research progress. While his career as a clinician, clinical scientist and medical trainee educator was thriving, this was a discouraging period. Nonetheless, Peter continued to publish papers on synaptic pruning during the five years after the 1979 publication. And he persisted with grant applications until he again procured NIH funding in 1985.

Over their many visits to Lausanne, Peter and Janellen became close friends with Hendrik and his family. In the acknowledgements section of his 2003 book *Neural Plasticity* [4], Peter wrote: "I would like to remember the late Hendrik Van der Loos, who stimulated my interest in developmental neurobiology and particularly my interest in neural plasticity. A key portion of my work on synaptogenesis was done during a sabbatical stay in the Institute of

Anatomy [in Lausanne] .... I miss him very much." As Janellen later wrote in an email, "Hendrick was a very attractive human and his wife was completely lovely. But it all ended so sadly." Hendrik died unexpectedly, by suicide, in the early 1990s after the death of his son. As Hendrik's wife wrote to Peter in November 1993 from Lausanne, Switzerland:

Dear Peter,

Thank you very much for your kind letter and for the positive words about Hendrik. We always remembered fondly our stay in Chicago and the discussion we had about families with growing children. It is sad to realize that our happy family of five now has dwindled to three, having to go on the strength of good memories.

Nolette

This loss had a big impact on Peter. Hendrik had enormous influence on Peter as a colleague, and as a friend.

With Hendrik, Peter studied synaptogenesis in the visual cortex. The visual cortex allowed for the precise measurement of cortical volume and addressed a key weakness of the 1979 study. Was the reduction in synapse density due to synapse elimination or alternatively due to an increase in total cortical volume? In this case they used computer-assisted methods for the quantification of synapses and area measurements. Their findings turned out to be similar to those made earlier regarding the prefrontal cortex [5]. There was an initial rapid increase in synaptic density and a subsequent decrease during later stages of development. However, the timing was different as both the burst of synapse density and subsequent synapse elimination took place earlier than in the prefrontal cortex, suggesting that not all brain regions show the same kinetics of synapse density over time. Crucially, the study showed that synaptic pruning occurs in different regions of the brain and is not limited to the prefrontal cortex.

Although the gap in funding was discouraging it was not terminal. With an influx of new NIH funding in 1985, Peter at age 54 embarked upon the next phase of his research – understanding synaptogenesis in different regions of the brain. In collaboration with a research assistant, Arun Dabholkar, he performed a developmental study that showed that different regions of the brain display distinct developmental time courses [6] (Figure 12.1). In Peter's personal collection, he had many images of neurons, hand drawn, showing specific morphologies and cell projections (Figure 12.2), and also included were data in his personal notebook that included the quantification of synapse density as a function of age in specific brain regions (Figure 12.3). In the

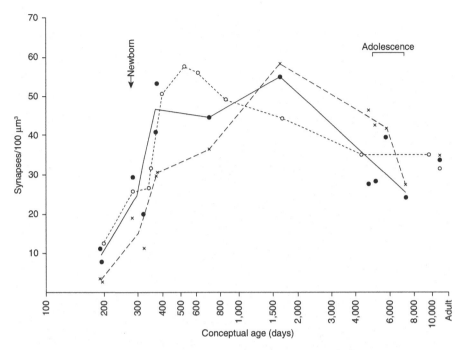

Figure 12.1 Mean synaptic density in synapses/100 micron area in the auditory, calcarine and prefrontal cortex at different ages. Open circles, visual cortex (area 17), filled circles, auditory cortex: crosses, prefrontal cortex (middle frontal gyrus). From: Huttenlocher PR, Dabholkar AS. 1997. Regional differences in synaptogenesis in human cerebral cortex. *J Comp Neurol* 387: 167–78. doi: 10.1002/(sici)1096-9861(19971020) 387:2<167::aid-cne1>3.0.co;2-z. Reprinted with permission.

primary visual cortex, maximum density is reached by eight months, whereas synaptogenesis in the middle prefrontal cortex develops later, with a peak in synaptic density at between three and four years of age. The data also suggested that synapse elimination occurred later in the middle frontal gyrus: at least until the early 20s, but due to some age gaps in the sample set, likely later. This is in contrast to the visual cortex, where adult levels of synaptic density may be reached as early as four years of age. The findings in the language areas particularly piqued Peter and Arun's interest. They found that the development of synapses in the auditory cortex, which controls hearing, preceded that in the "receptive" learning areas known as Wernicke's area. In addition, the development of synapses in Wernicke's area came before synaptogenesis in Broca's area, which controls motor speech. This elegantly supported the idea that the development of synapses mirrors the functional development of hearing sounds, then language comprehension and finally the ability to talk.

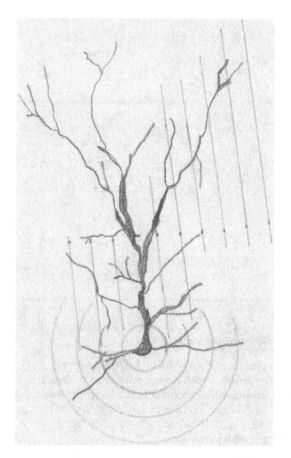

Figure 12.2 One of many pictures drawn by Peter of a neuron, imaged using the Golgi stain, to quantify the many projections that emanate from the cell body of the neuron. Personal collection.

In the concluding paragraph in their 1997 publication Huttenlocher and Dabholkar highlight the kinetics of synapse elimination in different regions of the brain, which correlate with later regression in regions that control higher cognitive functions:

> Onset of cortical function in the human appears to occur at different ages in different cortical regions. Functional development of prefrontal cortex appears to be more gradual and at a later age than visual cortex. . . . More complex "executive" functions of prefrontal cortex such as reasoning, motivation, and judgment appear to develop gradually during childhood and adolescence, perhaps continuing during the adult years. These uniquely human functions appear late during

Synaptic Density, entire Cortex.

Age	Syn/μ^2	syn/μ^3 $\left(=\dfrac{Syn}{\mu^2\times.0754}\right)$	Abercrombie corr Syn/mm^3 $\left(P=A\left(\dfrac{M}{L+M}\right)\times20\right)$	$\times10^8$
Gest. 28 wks	0.022	0.296	$(.296)\left(\dfrac{.075}{.284+.075}\right)\times20$	1.24
15 days	0.048	0.635	$(.635)\left(\dfrac{.075}{.302+.075}\right)\times20$	2.53
2 mo.	0.050	0.668	$(.668)\left(\dfrac{.075}{.377}\right)\times20$	2.66
2.5 mo.	0.060	0.796	$(.796)(.199)\times20$	3.17
4 mo.	0.095	1.27	$(1.27)\left(\dfrac{.075}{.377}\right)\times20$	5.05
8 mo.	0.115	1.53	$(1.53)\left(\dfrac{.075}{.326+.075}\right)\times20$	5.72
11 mo.	0.112	1.50	$(1.50)\left(\dfrac{.075}{.424}\right)\times20$	5.61
19 mo.	0.105	1.40	$(1.40)\left(\dfrac{.075}{.354+.075}\right)\times20$	4.90
3 4/12 yrs.	0.096	1.27	$(1.27)\left(\dfrac{.075}{.424}\right)\times20$	4.44
11 yrs.	0.076	1.01	$(1.01)(.35)$	3.54
26 yrs.	0.076	1.01	$(1.01)(.35)$	3.54
71 yrs.	0.0??	0.9??	$(.4??)(.35)$	3.??

Figure 12.3 From one of Peter's laboratory notebooks. Data showing the quantification of synapse density over age from a specific region of the brain. Note that the peak synapse density in this region of the brain is at 8–11 months of age with reduction by 19 months.

development, and their emergence may be aided by late persistence of exuberant synapses in the prefrontal cortex.

Like the studies in kittens by Hubel and Wiessel done in the 1960s, there was a window of time during which this synaptic remodeling occurred that reflected a time of significant plasticity. In humans, this "critical period" seemed to be prolonged as compared to other mammals. This window in humans is a time when learning occurs rapidly, and it makes sense that specific synaptic connections that are reinforced are sustained while others are lost. Peter's newer work suggested that this occurs at different times in different regions of the brain, correlating with the ages at which we learn and develop different skills. For example, the timing of pruning in the auditory cortex is consistent with the ease of learning a new language or music at a younger age. Peter was well aware of this gap since he had retained a thick German accent, even after having lived in the United States for many decades. Another example is the timing of pruning in the visual cortex corresponding with the developmental window seen with the reversal of amblyopia, or "lazy eye," by patching the strong eye and thereby forcing young children to use the weak eye.

As Irwin Feinberg noted, "science is a process of consensus-building." After the publication of Peter's 1979 paper there was a burst of work to address the pruning hypothesis in other animal models. Studies in primates, cats and mice all supported the idea that more connections are made early in development and that they are subsequently refined in an elegant process of selection. As discussed in Chapter 2, Shatz and colleagues showed that neural activity regulates synaptic pruning in the visual system of cats. Retinal cells in the eye send out exuberant branched projections and many of the connections are pruned away during development. However, if the retinal activity is blocked, the chaotic branches persist and are not pruned, providing direct evidence that neuronal activity regulates pruning in an elegant system that refines connections based on experience.

This work built upon years of prior neurobiology discoveries all the way back to the work of Ramón y Cajal almost a century earlier, and provided understanding for the developmental growth of neurons and their axon and dendrite projections as they reach out and touch neighboring cells. Some of these connections are sustained. Initial contacts between neurons seem to form in an organized way, but randomly. Based on activity or environmental input, specific synapses are then reinforced but, if the electrical and signaling activities do not occur in synapses, they are pruned or eliminated. It is a well-designed system: make too many and refine to select the optimal connections based on experience.

Scientific understanding of a biological phenomenon like synaptic pruning generally occurs over many decades, through a community process. Early in this process there is rarely a consensus and, often, much skepticism and disagreement. For Peter, the skeptics were difficult to handle because, more so than many scientists, he shied away from rancor, disagreement or making "waves," even though this is part of the scientific process. To him, his data clearly showed that there were regional differences in the kinetics of synapse loss, and that these regional differences correlated with the times of most intense learning in these different regions of the brain. This finding had broad implications for the relationship between synaptic pruning and learning and memory. There was debate in the field about the work in different regions of the brain. Work from Rakic and colleagues in primates suggested that the pruning did not show regional differences in synapse loss [7]. Peter thought this reflected the timing of pruning – that humans, with more complex processing such as spoken language and higher cognitive functions, had a more prolonged loss of synapses that extended through adolescence and even into adulthood. Indeed, in a more recent study published by Rakic and colleagues in 2011, with more human tissue samples, this is precisely what was found [8]. Elimination of synaptic spines in human brains extended into the third decade of life, supporting the idea of an extended period of "developmental reorganization."

Peter was excited to discuss plausible broader implications of the work focused on differential rates of synaptic pruning in different brain regions. In contrast to other animal species, the period of plasticity before synapse elimination is complete is much longer during human brain development. "There has been a great deal of emphasis lately on the importance of early learning," Dr. Huttenlocher said in a University of Chicago publication. He continued:

That is important, but we need to realize what children are able to learn and not cram them with information they are not ready to handle. Similarly, we need to appreciate what adolescents can learn. They are able to perform higher-level thinking that is beyond most younger children. We also need to realize that because the portion of the brain controlling motivation develops last, we shouldn't be surprised if high school students have trouble making decisions about their life's work. It may very well be that their brains need to develop further, that their brains simply aren't prepared to make such decisions until early adulthood.

References

1. P. R. Huttenlocher. Synaptic density in human frontal cortex: Developmental changes and effects of aging. *Brain Res.* 1979; **163**: 195–205.

2. J. P. Changeux and A. Danchin. Selective stabilization of developing synapses as a mechanism for the specification of neuronal networks. *Nature* 1976; **264**: 705–12.

3. M.E. Molliver, I. Kostovic and H. Van der Loos. The development of synapses in cerebral cortex of human fetus. *Brain Res* 1973; **50**: 403–7.

4. P. R. Huttenlocher. *Neural Plasticity: The Effects of Environment on the Development of the Cerebral Cortex*. Harvard University Press, 2002.

5. P.R. Huttenlocher, C. de Courten, L.J. Garey et al. Synaptogenesis in human visual cortex: Evidence for synapse elimination during normal development. *Neurosci Lett* 1982; **33**: 247–52.

6. P.R. Huttenlocher and A.S. Dabholkar. Regional differences in synaptogenesis in cerebral cortex. *J Comp Neurol* 1997; **387**: 167–78.

7. P. Rakic, J.P. Bourgeois, M.F. Eckenhoff et al. Concurrent overproduction of synapses in diverse regions of the primate cerebral cortex. *Science* 1986; **232**: 232–5.

8. Z. Petanjek, M. Judas, G. Simic et al. Extraordinary neoteny of synaptic spines in the human prefrontal cortex. *Proc Natl Acad Sci USA* 2011; **108**: 13281–6.

13 STIMULATING PROGRESS ON DEVELOPMENTAL BRAIN DISORDERS

Sometimes in science you experience an "aha" moment. It can happen while sitting in a talk, reading a paper, doing an experiment or doing the evening dishes. And when you have this jump in understanding it is hard to contain the thrill and excitement. Of course, you might be wrong – the next morning may reveal all the holes. But scientists cherish these infrequent moments when they make a new scientific connection that could change the way they – and subsequently others – think about a problem. This is precisely what happened in May 1993 when the young group leader Chris Walsh heard Peter Huttenlocher present at a neurology meeting focused on epilepsy in Venice, Italy.

Early on, Peter recognized the importance of having a clinic focused on developmental brain disorders. Many of these patients presented with symptoms that did not fit a specific condition or genetic disorder. Peter was especially interested in patients with tuberous sclerosis and related disorders, and examined brain tissue from families with these disorders using the "Golgi stain" (Figure 13.1). Tuberous sclerosis is a rare genetic condition associated with the formation of "tumors" or "tubers" in the brain. In Venice, Peter presented a talk about a family with a developmental brain disorder who he had seen through his tuberous sclerosis clinic at the University of Chicago. However, the family he described in Italy did not have tuberous sclerosis but rather had a kind of tuberous sclerosis mimic that was particularly interesting. Family members presented with seizures and had nodular subependymal masses of the brain by MRI scan. In this family there were six affected family members, all female, from four different generations. This was consistent with an X-linked dominant inheritance with a lack of survival in affected males. Periventricular heterotopia is the term used to describe the disorder of cortical brain development found in this family, characterized by neural cell masses along the lateral ventricles of the brain.

Chris Walsh was invited to the Venice meeting to present his work on cell lineage analysis in the developing brains of mice. Walsh was particularly interested in cell migration defects that lead to developmental disorders. As Walsh heard the description of this family in detail, he realized that he could "study this

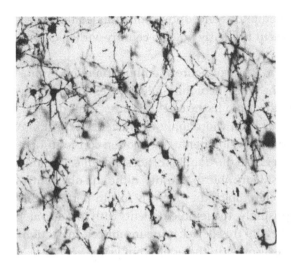

Figure 13.1 Image of small multipolar stellate neurons in a tuber from a patient with tuberous sclerosis. Personal collection.

family using brain scans to define anatomical abnormalities as a way of defining whether they were sick or not, and combining that with genetics." In a conversation in December 2021, Chris Walsh said, "This was just a pivotal moment, and my palms were sweating, my heart was racing when he was presenting it, and I just couldn't wait to talk to him and try to collaborate with him." Walsh said that this collaboration changed the trajectory of what was to become a highly successful research career. He became a geneticist. Instead of understanding the molecular mechanisms or pathogenesis of a disease first, the approach was to map and identify the genes and "understand mechanisms later."

The patients in the affected family had periventricular heterotopia, now confirmed as an X-linked dominant cause of "epilepsy" or seizure disorder. The patients had no evidence of developmental delay or other stigmata of disease. For Chris Walsh, this was a turning point in his science. It was the first gene he mapped, and he mapped it based on MRI findings. Walsh knew Peter from his training as a medical student at the University of Chicago. When he approached Peter at the meeting, he asked, "Would you like to collaborate to map the gene in this family?" Chris said that Peter looked "baffled" – and asked, "Map a gene?" This was before it was common to map genetic disorders, and the challenges were many. Walsh said that the four of them – Janellen, Peter, Chris Walsh and Chris' wife Ming Hui, also a scientist – went out to dinner in Venice and toasted to celebrate the new collaboration. DNA samples were sent and the gene was mapped in a few months, and published in the journal *Neuron* [1]. It was a serendipitous encounter that changed the trajectory of a career, but as Louis Pasteur famously noted a century earlier, chance favors the prepared mind.

During embryonic development, cortical neurons embark on a long-range directed migration from deep in the brain, near fluid-filled spaces known as the ventricles, to the outer region of the brain in the cerebral cortex. This developmental migration of neurons has been thoroughly characterized in mouse models. Perturbation of this normal developmental navigation can contribute to human developmental disorders like the double cortex syndrome. In many of these syndromes, the neurons still are able to migrate, although aberrantly. In the case of periventricular heterotopia, the neurons fail to perform this developmental migration. Surprisingly, the female patients with this disorder still have normal intelligence despite this defect in neuronal cell migration, and the presentation of a seizure disorder in the adolescent years.

It took the Walsh laboratory over five years to identify the gene responsible for "Huttenlocher's" classic X-linked bilateral form of periventricular heterotopia [2]. The gene was in a dense region of the genome and was a challenge to uncover. The responsible gene was identified as the *FLNA* gene that encodes the cytoskeletal protein filamin A. The cytoskeleton of the cell is a meshwork of membrane-associated proteins that provides structure to the cell. Its most abundant member is the cytoskeletal protein actin that polymerizes to form microfilaments. Dynamic regulation of the actin cytoskeleton is critical for cell movement. While doing the research for this book, as a physician scientist, I was particularly excited by the identification of filamin as the underlying etiology of periventricular heterotopia. My own research focuses on cell migration and how interactions between the matrix environment in tissues, outside of the cell, link to the cytoskeleton inside the cell to control cell migration. In prior work, we and others had found that the strength of these linkages between cell surface adhesion receptors – integrins – and the cytoskeleton play a key role in controlling cell migration.

Filamin is a cytoskeletal protein that links cell surface adhesion receptors to the actin cytoskeleton. This critical connection enables the appropriate amount of adhesion of a cell to the surrounding extracellular environment to allow cells to migrate the right amount – not too much and not too little. Filamin provides a linkage that allows the cell to sense its outside environment, the matrix tissue in which the cells navigate and move. Without these connections between the cell surface receptors and the intracellular cytoskeletal machinery, cell movement is not possible. Due to the point mutations found in patients with periventricular heterotopia, the function of filamin is disabled. The Walsh group's study was the first to show that filamin plays a critical role in neuronal cell migration. It is a classic story of a basic biomedical science discovery. One physician scientist was sufficiently alert to identify a patient family with an apparently heritable defect, and sufficiently curious to define some of the resulting tissue defects underpinning the disease. A second physician scientist heard them talk at a meeting and was sufficiently insightful to prioritize investigating the matter for multiple years, and sufficiently talented to identify the causal gene and reveal a previously unknown core mechanism involved in brain development.

The finding that filamin plays a role in neuronal cell migration was unexpected. It is an example of how genetic analysis often uncovers new biochemical or cellular functions. Sometimes this type of discovery launches entire new fields by uncovering new functions and signaling networks. It was already known that filamin regulates the cytoskeleton in leukocytes, but this was the first evidence that it regulates neuronal migration. In this case, although the discovery revealed a neuronal mechanism and provided an explanation for a genetic syndrome, it has not yet led to new treatments. This gap between understanding a malady and learning how to intervene and treat a disease is a common "next challenge" in biomedical research.

These types of cases are the ultimate motivation for physician scientists. Can we make discoveries that affect the treatment and outcome for our patients? Chris Walsh is now a global leader whose research group has used genetics to uncover the causes of many other human neurodevelopmental disorders. In a recent interview published in the journal *PNAS* [3], he noted that more recently he has been switching his focus to understand even more about the "basic biology" that regulates human brain development. He is in good company as a physician scientist whose medical training has helped him excel at uncovering important molecular mechanisms – the foundational knowledge – rather than focusing on the development of disease treatments or other applications of that knowledge.

References

1. Y. Z. Eksioglu, I. E. Scheffer, P. Cardenas et al. Periventricular heterotopia: An X-linked dominant epilepsy locus causing aberrant cerebral cortical development. *Neuron* 1996; **16**: 77–87.
2. J. W. Fox, E. D. Lamperti, Y. Z. Eksioglu et al. Mutations in filamin 1 prevent migration of cerebral cortical neurons in human periventricular heterotopia. *Neuron* 1998; **21**: 1315–25.
3. S. Ravindran. Profile of Chris Walsh. *Proc Natl Acad USA* 2020; **117**: 13861–63.

14 NEURODEVELOPMENTAL DISORDERS AND SCHIZOPHRENIA: A ROLE FOR SYNAPTIC PRUNING?

The beauty of Peter's work is that he mapped what happened in the brain after birth. There were data on what happens before birth, but more happens after birth than we had ever imagined. It explains why no child can recollect memories before 2 years of age – there are too many connections; it is a cacophony and the symphony has not yet started.

Huda Zoghbi, Professor, Baylor College of Medicine, 2019

Huda Zoghbi is an expert on the genetics of neurodevelopmental disease. Zoghbi and her research group uncovered the genetic basis of a classic postnatal neurodevelopmental disorder, Rett syndrome. It is a puzzling disorder in girls who develop normally for the first year of life or more – reaching milestones like walking and talking – and then undergo a regression at around one to two years of age. The developmental deterioration coincides with the timing when there is a switch from net synapse formation to synapse elimination. As a medical resident, Zoghbi became fascinated with understanding what is happening in Rett syndrome. Zoghbi initially described a cohort of girls published in the *New England Journal of Medicine* in 1985 and proposed a genetic etiology on the X chromosome [1]. Years later, after receiving training in genetics, Zoghbi returned to Rett syndrome and uncovered its genetic cause. Rett syndrome is an X-linked dominant disorder due to mutations in the methyl-CpG-binding protein 2 (MeCP2), which is encoded by the gene *MeCP2* [2]. Zoghbi's more recent work in mouse models has shown that the MeCP2 overabundance leads to increased synapse density and autistic-like behaviors, suggesting a dose-dependent effect of MeCP2 levels on outcome. This is in accordance with the finding that humans with gene duplications in the *MeCP2* gene have autism spectrum disorder (referred to herein as autism). It is less clear if there is in fact a direct connection between MeCP2 and synaptic pruning. However, recent studies suggest that mutations in the *MeCP2* gene may lead to age-related defects in synapse pruning in the first year of life. Indeed, work from the group of Beth Stevens has suggested that MeCP2 deficiency in mice weakens synapses, making them more susceptible to pruning and removal by microglial cells [3].

Peter Huttenlocher's early work on synaptic pruning was largely observational or descriptive. During conversations in March 2019, Zoghbi said: "Observational science is important, but it is hard to get funded. Peter was ahead of the time – he made the human discovery before the disease part was in place." She continued, "No one thought that the babies are born with the hardware largely intact, and the key process to development after birth is to refine synapses and select which ones will be functional. No one imagined it was at the root of so many disorders." A key distinguishing feature of many neurodevelopmental disorders is that they are postnatal diseases, as compared to the neuronal migration disorders that have origin early in prenatal development. Neurodevelopmental disorders include autism and attention-deficit/hyperactivity disorder. Even diseases with later onset in adolescence or young adulthood, like schizophrenia, are now considered to be neurodevelopmental disorders. Increasing evidence suggests a link between aberrant synaptic pruning in childhood and neurodevelopmental disorders. But many gaps and challenges remain. Human brains are different from animal models and are difficult to study over time. The ability to image synapses in humans as children develop remains a major challenge. Zoghbi noted: "This requires a non-invasive way to look at connections, using synaptic tracers to quantify synapse numbers in living humans."

Despite these challenges, growing evidence supports a connection between neurodevelopmental disease and defects in pruning, either too much or too little pruning, which impact brain circuitry in different regions of the brain. For example, with autism, there is evidence to suggest that there is a surplus of synapses that contribute to a "cacophony" in the brain. This affects normal development and social interactions, often with onset at the time of robust pruning, before three years of age. Autism is a heterogeneous disorder with different symptoms across patients; however, syndromic autism, like Rett syndrome, provides a way to get at the genetic basis for some types of autism. This type of progress has been essential to provide further insight into the connection between autism and synaptic pruning, by categorizing the different types of autism.

Evidence to support a defect in synaptic pruning in autism has been provided by observations of post-mortem brain samples, showing increased dendritic spine density in patients with autism. Some forms of autism are due to mutations in pathways that affect a protein kinase known as mammalian target of rapamycin (mTOR) [4]. Mouse models of these gene variants also show a surplus of synapses, and this effect can be abrogated by inhibiting this pathway using a drug known as rapamycin, an immunosuppressant. Indeed, clinical trials are ongoing to test the effects of rapamycin on the development of autism in patients with tuberous sclerosis. It is an intriguing idea that increasing synaptic pruning early on may improve the prognosis in patients who will develop autism.

Schizophrenia is a neurodevelopmental disorder with a later onset than autism, after the most robust early synaptic pruning has occurred in young children. However, schizophrenia is thought to be a disorder associated with too much pruning in regions of the brain involved in higher cognitive functions. These regions are pruned later in development, with pruning continuing into adolescence and early adulthood, the time when many individuals are diagnosed with schizophrenia. It is also likely that schizophrenia is multifactorial, combining genetic susceptibility, environmental factors and a connectivity problem. Schizophrenia is unlike autism spectrum disorders, which have an early age of onset during a critical period of synapse elimination.

The idea that synaptic pruning may be part of schizophrenia was first proposed by the psychiatrist Irwin Feinberg. As noted in Chapter 9, Feinberg was a postdoctoral fellow in the same laboratory as Peter at the National Institutes of Health (NIH). They remained in contact after leaving NIH and Feinberg was influenced by Peter's findings of developmental synaptic pruning. He was particularly intrigued by the data suggesting that synaptic pruning may extend through adolescence in regions of the brain associated with higher cognitive functions. For Feinberg, reading Peter's previously mentioned landmark 1979 paper in *Brain Research* provided a clue to a problem that had puzzled him: Why was there regressive change in REM (rapid eye movement) sleep over adolescence? Feinberg had previously reported age-related changes in EEG sleep patterns with a biphasic dependence of EEG wave amplitude during sleep as a function of age [5]. There was a peak in amplitude in childhood and a subsequent decline in adolescence and early adulthood (Figure 14.1), similar to the patterns in synapse elimination Peter reported in the frontal lobe during child development. The idea that all of this is happening at the same time helped Feinberg make the connection between sleep and synaptic pruning, and its potential role in schizophrenia.

As Feinberg went on to say during a conversation in May 2022, "sleep is deranged in schizophrenia – no characteristic sleep pattern – but it is disrupted." In 1983, Feinberg hypothesized that schizophrenia is a defect in

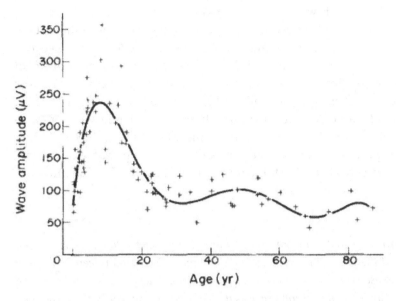

Figure 14.1 EEG sleep patterns as a function of age. Note peak sleep wave amplitude in early childhood and reduction with age, reminiscent of the reduction of synapse number with age. From Feinberg I. Schizophrenia: Caused by a fault in programmed synaptic elimination during adolescence? *J Psychiatr Res* 1982; 17: 319–34. Reprinted with permission.

programmed synaptic elimination during adolescence. He published this idea in the *Journal of Psychiatric Research* [6]:

> *Converging evidence indicates that a profound reorganization of human brain function takes place during adolescence . . . . A reduction in cortical synaptic density has recently been observed and may account for all of these changes . . . . Such synaptic "pruning" may be analogous to the programmed elimination of neural elements in very early development. A defect in this maturational process may underlie those cases of schizophrenia that emerge during adolescence.*

Feinberg hypothesized that these changes occur when there is a known reduction in brain metabolism and deep sleep during adolescence. Seth Cohen, a former trainee of Feinberg's in Psychiatry at UCSF, wrote in an email in November 2018: "Your father's work had a very significant influence on Dr. Feinberg's thinking." Based on the observation of developmental synaptic elimination, Feinberg proposed that schizophrenia was, in essence, a disorder of synaptic pruning gone "awry." It is possible that the wrong synapses are eliminated in schizophrenia, or that too many synapses are eliminated.

Feinberg's hypothesis was largely ignored at the time. Decades later, work by Steve Carroll and Beth Stevens has suggested a genetic basis to support the pruning hypothesis in schizophrenia [7]. This proposed relationship between schizophrenia and synapse elimination was, according to Feinberg, "ahead of its time and did not have a framework to exist in." Feinberg went on: "There is resistance to new ideas in science without being backed up with data." At that time, it was "all about dopamine in schizophrenia" – and there was not much interest in other ideas. This situation with schizophrenia is similar to that for the synaptic pruning discovery more broadly: a finding that was decades ahead of its time, and we are still learning the full extent of its meaning for normal development or disease.

Feinberg said:

I might have ignored it – but I knew Huttenlocher was a meticulous researcher, and it explained the change in sleep during this time – decrease in deep wave sleep during adolescence with massive changes of brain metabolic rate – profound reorganization of brain during adolescence. It made sense, cut back on the ones that are not successfully integrated. If you have such a massive change – it may sometimes be imperfect. If there are errors – too many or too few – mental illness may result. Age of onset of schizophrenia – often at the ends of adolescence and early 20s. Reduction in deep sleep – REM sleep in schizophrenia/reduction of prefrontal cortex of new membrane – whatever normally happens during adolescence is exaggerated in schizophrenia – there is more reduction.

Feinberg said his talk at the Society of Neuroscience meeting in the 1980s proposing the synaptic pruning hypothesis in schizophrenia seemed to have been largely ignored. However, the next day, another neuroscientist and "a bit of 'a hustler,' who worked in the field of synapse remodeling, raised a similar concept in his talk – as though it was his idea – even though he had never done anything in schizophrenia." Feinberg was flabbergasted and said: "Now, I may have made more of an issue, but it just turned me off. This was someone who usurped other's achievements – and I distrusted him. I just moved on." This aspect of science – the element of competition and lack of generosity to colleagues – had significantly repelled both Peter and Feinberg so many years ago, as young scientists training at NIH. Their approach was to just move on and not raise a fuss. However, it is important to consider that the quieter, more modest scientists who think differently, like Peter and Irwin, are often overlooked or even ignored for years, and that this can slow down the pace of scientific breakthroughs and innovation. It may be productive to more explicitly train reticent scientists in skills such as scientific debate, networking and career advancement. It also is critical to recognize and promote different types of scientists or approaches that contribute in their own unique ways to pushing fields forward.

Thirty-five years after Feinberg first proposed a link between schizophrenia and abnormal synaptic pruning, genetic evidence has provided direct support for this idea. The findings involve the complement system made up of a few dozen plasma proteins, which work with the immune system to protect against infections and to remove dead cells and foreign material. Work from Steve Carroll's laboratory at the Broad Institute and the Stevens Laboratory at Harvard has shown that the complement *C4* gene is linked to schizophrenia risk (see also Chapter 17 on microglial cells and pruning) [7]. They found an association between increased *C4* expression and increased risk for schizophrenia. This work provided a possible explanation for the increase in synaptic pruning in schizophrenia through the action of microglia-mediated elimination, a process that is regulated by complement components. In addition to the genetic link, recent human post-mortem brain studies also support the hypothesis that synapses are over-pruned in schizophrenia. Golgi staining from autopsy samples show that individuals with schizophrenia have reduced dendritic spine density in the cerebral cortex as compared to age-matched controls [8]. Taken together, these studies provide a strong link between synaptic pruning gone awry and the development of schizophrenia. However, challenges remain before this theory gains full acceptance.

Although post-mortem studies are consistent with the "over-pruning hypothesis," they provide only one snapshot in time. How do synapse number and function change in the same individual over time? How is this different in an adolescent child who goes on to develop schizophrenia? The challenge is to understand how synapses change over time during adolescence and how this is altered in individuals who end up developing schizophrenia. And, ultimately, to discover if interventions – drugs or other treatments – alter this pruning phenotype and treat schizophrenia.

The window into understanding synapses in the human brain has been improving with advances in brain imaging techniques. Previous imaging studies had shown increased cortical thinning in people who develop schizophrenia, also supporting the over-pruning hypothesis in schizophrenia [9]. However, the advent of a more refined imaging of synapses using PET scanning is allowing even more insight into how synapses change in humans over time. The development of the PET tracer [^{11}C]UCB to image the synapse marker SV2A has been used to show that in patients with advanced schizophrenia there is reduced binding of the synapse marker, suggesting that these individuals have over-pruning of their synapses [10]. There are caveats, however. It is unclear if this reduction represents actual pruning or if these synapses remain intact but are just less functional or less active. In addition, this work was done with patients with advanced disease, rather than new-onset schizophrenia. It is this challenge that physician scientist Jong Yoon, Professor at Stanford University, is grappling with.

In an interview with Jong Yoon in May 2022, he said that "Feinberg is usually very critical – but, with Peter, he was always very laudatory of Peter's work." Yoon said that looking at markers of synapses in patients provides a more "distal product to test the pruning hypothesis." He is studying schizophrenia patients early in their disease course to address the chicken or egg question: what comes first – the disease or the over-pruning? In unpublished findings, Yoon has found a dramatic difference with excessive pruning early in schizophrenia – suggesting that it is an early step in disease pathogenesis. Yoon noted that usually there are messy results in schizophrenia research because schizophrenia is a heterogenous disorder – meaning many different underlying causes contribute to disease – including distinct genetic factors and environmental triggers. But with the pruning studies early in schizophrenia, "the results are clean and occur in wide regions of the brain." This is an exciting advance that further implicates abnormal pruning in schizophrenia. The next step is to refine these studies – and look earlier before the onset of disease in families with a high risk for developing schizophrenia. And, ultimately, to intervene by treating patients with drugs that target pruning – complement inhibitors, for example, that alter the microglia-mediated elimination of synapses. Do these treatments alter synapses by brain imaging and alter the course of disease? Pharmaceutical companies have taken note. These types of interventions are in the works and have entered clinical trials for psychiatric disease.

Recent studies with human *in vitro* models (cells in a dish), using inducible pluripotent stem cells from patients with schizophrenia, also support the idea of increased complement-mediated synapse elimination by microglial cells [11]. This provides a particularly useful tool for drug discovery, and in this recent work the authors found that the antibiotic minocycline reduces microglia-mediated synapse engulfment. In addition, based on medical record reviews, it has been found that patients treated with minocycline had a modest reduction in risk for developing schizophrenia. In any case, this type of human *in vitro* model will provide a powerful tool for future studies of synaptic pruning and how it is altered in specific diseases like schizophrenia.

The idea that aberrant synaptic pruning provides a potentially targetable pathology is in its infancy but also extremely exciting. The neurodevelopmental disorders span multiple disorders of childhood including autism and schizophrenia, which commonly arises in late adolescence or early adulthood. These are among the more prominent neurologic disorders in human medicine, but many questions remain. In the decades since the first discovery of synaptic pruning more questions than answers have emerged, challenging scientists to continue their hunt for new discoveries.

References

1. H. Y. Zoghbi, A.K. Percy, D.G. Glaze et al. Reduction of biogenic amine levels in the Rett syndrome. *N Engl J Med* 1985; **313**: 921–4.
2. R. E. Amir, I.B. Van den Veyver, M. Wan et al. Rett syndrome is caused by mutations in X-linked *MECP2*, encoding methyl-CpG binding protein 2. *Nat Genet* 1999; **23**: 185–88.
3. D. P. Schafer, C.T. Heller, G. Gunner et al. Microglia contribute to circuit defects in Mecp2 null mice independent of microglia-specific loss of Mecp2 expression. *ELife* 2016; **5**: e15224.
4. G. Tang, K. Gudsnuk, S.H. Kuo et al. Loss of mTOR-dependent macroauto-phagy causes autistic-like synaptic pruning deficits. *Neuron* 2014; **83**: 1131–43.
5. I. Feinberg, R.L. Koresko and N. Heller. EEG patterns as a function of normal and pathological aging in man. *J Psychiatr Res* 1967; **5**: 107–44.
6. I. Feinberg. Schizophrenia: Caused by a fault in programmed synaptic elimination during adolescence? *J Psychiatr Res* 1982; **17**: 319–34.
7. A. Sekar, A. R. Bialas, H. de Rivera H et al. Schizophrenia risk from complex variation of complement component 4. *Nature* 2016; **530**: 177–83.
8. B. van Berlekom, C. H. Muflihah, G. J. L. J. Snijders et al. Synapse pathology in schizophrenia: A meta-analysis of postsynaptic elements in postmortem brain studies. *Schizophr Bull* 2020; **46**: 374–86.
9. T. D. Cannon, Y. Chung, G. He et al. Progressive reduction in cortical thickness as psychosis develops: A multisite longitudinal neuroimaging study of youth at elevated risk. *Biol Psychiatry* 2015: **77**: 147–57.
10. E. C. Onwordi, E. F. Halff, T. Whitehurst, et al. Synaptic density marker SV2A is reduced in schizophrenia patients and unaffected by antipsychotics in rats. *Nat Commun* 2020; 11: 246.
11. C. M. Sellgren, J. Gracias, B. Watmuff et al. Increased synapse elimination by microglia in schizophrenia patient-derived models of synaptic pruning. *Nat Neurosci* 2019; **22**: 374–85.

15 EARLY CHILDHOOD EDUCATION

Neurons that fire together wire together.
LEARN Behavioral website: Brain Plasticity and Early Intervention

The concept of synaptic pruning had an impact on mainstream thinking about early education soon after its discovery. The fact that millions of synapses are eliminated between early childhood and adulthood was mind boggling. But conceptually, it made sense that the brain circuitry starts with more connections than are needed, and subsequently can be sculpted based on input. Although it may seem inefficient, the early overabundance of connections enables a process for selective elimination and refinement that occurs over years, as children learn. But how does synaptic pruning relate to childhood learning? Education scholars and advocates had for centuries been alert to the positive impacts of education on child development. In 1979, education initiatives such as the Head Start program in the United States were already in place. The discovery of synaptic pruning then supplied a new and specific biological basis supporting the benefits of early childhood education.

Discoveries about synaptic pruning and brain plasticity helped to set in motion a new wave of proposals for educational interventions to, in essence, "train the brain." The idea of brain plasticity also triggered a flurry of articles in the popular press in the 1990s, in *Newsweek*, *Time*, *US News* and *World Report* and other venues, with titles like "Brain talk" or "How a child's brain develops." The *New York Times* reported in an obituary in August 2013 that Peter's findings had "influenced education and government policy and parents' priorities, putting increased emphasis on the importance of early education. Today, parents of infants and toddlers encourage bilingualism or violin lessons at what they hope will be peak synaptic moments, school systems focus more on kindergarten and pre-kindergarten programs, and aging baby boomers download Sudoku apps in an effort to preserve precious neurons."

These ideas for how to educate young children were not without controversy. Is there in fact a "critical window for learning"? The idea that emerged during this time was to "teach children young so your child has more synapses!" Why do young children have increased capacity to learn and recover language after brain injury? Why do young children learn a second language easily, and without an accent? There is substantial evidence to support a kind of critical window that correlates with pruning in primary sensory regions of the brain, the areas that regulate hearing and vision and are associated with language acquisition. The development of musical ability, like language, is also an early process, for example in the association of perfect pitch with early exposure to music.

Plasticity in the development of language is a particularly intriguing area, since having advanced language skills is a process that in the words of Peter Huttenlocher is "uniquely human." And, accordingly, language processing in the brain is complex. "Within the human species, we find little evidence for a circumscribed language organ. The whole brain participates in language . . .," said Elizabeth Bates in 1993, as quoted in Peter's book *Neural Plasticity* [1]. However, specific regions of the brain had been implicated in language development, as early as the mid-1800s, based on studies of patients with unilateral brain injuries. In 1861, Paul Broca reported a Parisian shoemaker who had suffered a stroke previously and retained the ability to understand but was unable to speak or write due to a lesion in what became known as "Broca's area" in the frontal lobe. In 1879, Carl Wernicke described patients that retained the ability to speak but were unable to understand language due to lesions on the left back side of the brain, in an area now referred to as Wernicke's area. This supported the idea that regions of the brain had specialized functions in language. What is particularly interesting is what happens if these unilateral brain injuries occur earlier in life, during a period of substantial plasticity or capability for pruning and refining synapses. In contrast to adults with brain injuries in areas that mediate language and result in the inability to speak or understand language (aphasia), lesions in the same region of the brain of infants or young children often do not lead to significant language deficits. Peter's collaborator Susan Levine said, in an interview in February 2022, "it is shocking how well kids can do after brain injury to regions that affect language."

As Peter stated in *Neural Plasticity*: "There appears to be universal agreement language functions after focal injury such as stroke in infancy are remarkably different from those after stroke in the adult" [1]. Focal brain lesions in infants prior to the onset of language are not associated with aphasia or language deficits later in life, although there can be some delay in language development. The recovery is remarkable as compared to adult brain injuries. This is due to the significant brain plasticity in young children and represents a "window" in development when there is a high potential for recovery after injury. Later in Peter's career he became particularly interested in studying the brains of children after injury to further dissect brain plasticity and the potential for recovery using functional MRI. This work was funded as part of a large National Institutes of Health program project grant on longitudinal language on which Janellen served as the overall principal investigator. Peter's component of the grant was focused on using functional MRI to image the brains of children and to study the impact of brain injury in young children in collaboration with Susan Levine.

Despite clear evidence for early plasticity and the potential for learning during this time even after brain injury, the skeptics were many, including Peter himself. Are the first three years of life, when there is robust synaptic remodeling, important for long-term learning? Peter often noted that "more synapses or a density of synapses in the brain does not mean someone is smarter"; more is not necessarily better. Peter also believed that most types of learning continue throughout life and are not limited to specific early developmental windows. Bruer wrote in a critical commentary in *Nature Neuroscience* in 2002, "Peter Huttenlocher's work on changes in synaptic density over the life span has been prominent in media, policy and education articles" to support early intervention [2]. Bruer referenced other scientists who similarly suggested the importance of early education and its relationship to brain plasticity. But Bruer then wrote: "Unfortunately, in each case, it is the spurious, throwaway speculation, not the sound scientific result, that has captured the public's attention." Bruer did not think brain science should be applied to education and child development and referred to it as the "pediatrician's error." Peter, normally quiet in dissent, countered with a response, also published in *Nature Neuroscience* [3]. Although Peter agreed that learning continues throughout life, he argued that more science was needed to connect brain science and an understanding of how to optimize education experiences for young children. Peter wrote: "Old borders between disciplines are rapidly disappearing, in large part driven by new methods of investigation such as functional magnetic resonance imaging (fMRI). Examples of neuroscience data with practical implications are on the increase." He went on to say, "Bruer ridicules early intervention. Yet, many recent studies show that early education programs, begun before children are two years old, carry long-lasting benefits in selected populations, including disadvantaged and prematurely born infants."

Peter and his wife Janellen had long since wedded their passions for understanding brain plasticity and the role of the environment in child development and learning. In the above commentary, Peter noted, "The interface between developmental neuroscience and child development is an exciting area of investigation, driven by new technologies such as functional imaging. Collaboration between neuroscientists, developmental psychologists and educators will best advance this field."

References

1. P. R. Huttenlocher. *Neural Plasticity: The Effects of Environment on the Development of the Cerebral Cortex.* Harvard University Press, 2002.
2. J. T. Bruer. Avoiding the pediatricians error: How neuroscientists can help educators (and themselves). *Nat Neurosci* 2002; **5(suppl.)**: 1031–3.
3. P. R. Huttenlocher. Basic neuroscience research has important implictions for child development. *Nat Neurosci* 2003; **6**: 541.

16 PETER AND JANELLEN'S COLLABORATION

Peter and Janellen had shared ideas throughout their careers, molding each other's perspectives on the fields of brain plasticity and development. Their shared interest and distinct approaches were accurately highlighted when they were introduced to their new retirement community in the early 2000s, through the Montgomery Place newsletter.

> *Their professional interests overlap, and they have published joint papers. Peter is interested in the early development of the human brain, "Did you know that a baby has far more synapses than an adult? They have to be pruned." Janellen's field is cognitive and developmental psychology, and she is interested in how language and mathematical skills develop in children and the environmental effects on their development. Janellen says she is absorbed in her work. Peter is interested in music and in expressionist art.*

Although Peter and Janellen conversed extensively with each other about their work, they only published two manuscripts together. A 1973 paper described the first cohort of children with hyperlexia, a puzzling developmental condition associated with advanced reading skills in children who otherwise had impaired cognitive development [1]. A second collaborative manuscript was published in 1990, demonstrating that specific neurological tests in preschool children could predict subsequent developmental delay. It was proposed that this screening platform could be used to identify at-risk children who would benefit from early intervention programs [2]. An image of Peter and Janellen in Janellen's child development laboratory was taken as part of their collaboration (Figure 16.1).

Although they did not generally publish together, Peter's work on developmental pruning influenced Janellen's interest in the impact of the environment on learning. As part of a set of groundbreaking studies, Janellen's group recorded interactions between mothers and their children in Chicago and found that the language environment influenced children's vocabulary and syntax acquisition [3]. The studies showed that preschool children benefit

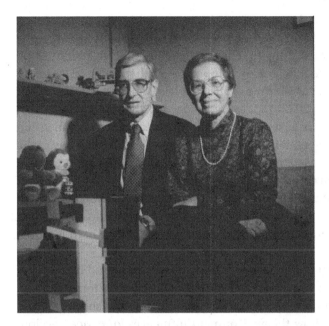

Figure 16.1 Peter and Janellen in Janellen's cognitive psychology laboratory at the University of Chicago.

when their parents and teachers use complex sentences in their conversations with children. This type of exposure increases the child's comprehension ability and subsequent vocabulary and use of complex sentences. In a related study, Janellen's research group found that children's ability to learn fluctuated depending on whether they were in school or out of school during the summer. This important work separated environment and genetic factors and provided direct evidence that environmental input affects language development. This work has been cited in studies suggesting that children would benefit from year-round schooling.

These studies by Janellen and her colleagues challenged a dogma in the field that had suggested that the organization of words into sentences, otherwise known as syntax, was developed naturally due to inborn traits that were programmed into the brain, rather than being influenced by the environment. Classic work by Noam Chomsky suggested that language is an innate ability and that children are born with a "universal grammar" that is inborn. In contrast, Janellen's studies suggested that language and grammar are learned and influenced by the environment in which children develop. Her work indicated that young children benefit from language-rich preschool classes – indeed, studies showed that young children experience a two-fold increase in the ability to form complex sentences in these kinds of environments. Janellen's work suggested that children need input, and benefit from it early. One concept that emerged from Janellen's studies is that vocabulary and language acquisition are different as compared to other types of learning, like spatial learning. Or, as Susan Levine, a colleague at the University of Chicago, said in February 2022: "not everything works the same way."

At the same time that Janellen was testing the effects of environment on child language development, Bill Greenough, a professor of psychology at the University of Illinois, provided compelling evidence showing the importance of experience and enriched environments for synapse formation in the brains of mammals, including later in life. His work showed that environmental enrichment, exercise and learning led to the development of new synapses in rodent models, further supporting the importance of environment on both learning and brain plasticity [4].

Susan Levine noted that "Janellen was a big ideas person and had a lot of influence because of that. Janellen understood that both innate factors (genetics) and environment influence cognitive development, but she wanted to understand more about how the environment influences language development, because you can do something about the environment." Levine went on to say that "Janellen was a giant in the field" with a lasting impact on understanding spatial thinking and language development. Kelly Mix, a former graduate student of Janellen's, and now a professor at the University of Maryland, commented that "Janellen would always say 'We came for the truth.' I learned so much from watching how she thought about things, how she tackled problems. She didn't want the data to support what she already was thinking, but rather, reveal what was actually happening."

Janellen was driven by research; she would spend hours at any time of the day or night scribbling on yellow lined sheets of paper – thinking, writing, refining, with glee. She was intense and focused, and loved what she did. It was hard to be a leader of your discipline and it was the determined few who did so. Susan Levine also noted that Janellen was "not political" and was not afraid to say what she thought. She was keenly critical. "Janellen made waves." Peter was the opposite; he did not make waves; he avoided conflict or self-promotion and so, as Levine said, "he often did not get the recognition he deserved." When Janellen or anyone else made waves Peter cringed in silence, not unlike his response to the bigwigs in science who were adept at promoting their work. While Janellen scribbled on her yellow note pads and worked, Peter often happily tinkered in his garden with his roses, strawberries, tomatoes or peach trees. Or with a self-constructed model train village or building a dollhouse for his children and grandchildren, listening to and reading about classical music or expressionist art or reading German literature or plays. He relished making a German plum or peach tart, playing the flute and writing program notes for the local youth orchestra performance. Peter's interests were broad. Janellen's interests were focused, although she enjoyed reading history and literature, and loved a good debate. Peter tried many different things, "and he was not into resume building." He was interested in doing what interested him. As Susan Levine went on to say, "He was deeply interested in the development of the human brain, but he had other interests as well." Levine pondered and ended by saying, "Peter was a renaissance man," and then, regarding Peter more generally, "Peter's was a story of resilience."

Although Peter's story was one of resilience and not making "waves," even years after having left Nazi Germany behind he bristled at authority. Occasionally, he more than bristled. One extreme example of this was an encounter with the City of Chicago police. As Janellen told the story, on an afternoon drive through the south side of Chicago, Peter was stopped by the police for failing to come to a complete stop at a stop sign. Peter denied it and retorted, "I did not go through the stop sign." He resisted. It escalated. Before Janellen was able to intervene, the police pulled Peter out of the car and roughly slammed him against the side of the car – and then frisked and handcuffed him. He was thrown into a police wagon; Peter, the gentle pediatric neurologist. Janellen followed the police wagon to the station, where she negotiated his release and "bailed him" out of jail. That the calm Dr. Huttenlocher had some-what forcefully resisted authority was not denied by the doctor himself, whose face would adopt a smug air of rebellion when the story was told at his expense.

Shortly after Peter's passing, I received the following email about a named lectureship in his honor from a scientific society focused on cognitive neuroscience, a field that bridges both Janellen's and Peter's work.

Dear Dr. Huttenlocher,

Our deepest sympathy on the passing of your father Dr. Peter Huttenlocher. The field has been very much stricken by his passing and we, collectively, have been discussing the importance of his pioneering contributions to the field. We are contacting you to let you know that the Scientific Program Committee of Flux: The International Congress for Integrative Developmental Cognitive Neuroscience has voted to name our Keynote Talk the "Huttenlocher Lecture" in his honor as **the father of Developmental Cognitive Neuroscience**. The "Huttenlocher Lecture" will be our feature plenary talk in all subsequent meetings. Our research has been significantly influenced by your father's pioneering work as evidenced by how we all cite his work in our publications. We are humbled at the opportunity to honor his memory. We both had the honor of meeting your father and were very impressed at how humble and generous he was in interacting with us. One of us (Bea) recently presented some of his work for the Institute of Medicine at the National Academy of Sciences to instruct policy about the protracted nature of neural development so he had been very much in my mind. One of us (Brad) is a pediatric neurologist who understands your father's tremendous contributions to that discipline as a physician, teacher, scientist, and mentor.

Best Regards,

Beatriz Luna Chair and Brad Schlaggar, Co-ChairFlux: The International Congress for Integrative Developmental Cognitive Neuroscience

A subsequent email to Janellen highlights the close relationship between Peter's and Janellen's research. Janellen described Mike Posner as "a brilliant and famous neuroscientist."

Dear Janellen,

I am not sure whether or not you know but this year I had the honor of being asked to deliver the Huttenlocher lecture during the FLUX meeting in St. Louis. It is great honor for me because while I did not know Peter, I do know you and I recognize that the two of you do span all that I love about connecting cognitive and brain science in development.

I want you to know that I will be thinking about you as well as Peter in September.

Mike Posner, Professor, University of Oregon

Janellen's long-term friend summed up Peter and Janellen's relationship, both on the intellectual and personal level: "You walked into a storybook marriage."

References

1. P. R. Huttenlocher and J. Huttenlocher. A study of children with hyperlexia. *Neurology* 1973; **23**: 1107–16.
2. P. R. Huttenlocher, S. C. Levine, J. Huttenlocher et al. Discrimination of normal and at risk preschool children on the basis of neurological tests. *Dev Med Child Neurol* 1990; **32**: 394–402.
3. J. Huttenlocher. Language input and language growth. *Prev Med* 1998; **27**: 195–99.
4. K. D. Federmeier, J. A. Kleim and W. T. Greenough. Learning-induced multiple synapse formation in rat cerebellar cortex. *Neurosci Lett* 2002; **332**: 180–84.

17 MICROGLIAL CELLS AND THE MECHANISMS OF SYNAPTIC PRUNING

The scientist must concern himself with what one will say about him in a century, rather than with current insults or compliments.

Louis Pasteur, French chemist (1822–1895)

In 1937, the Spanish neuroscientist and artist Ramón y Cajal commented on an apparent trial and error period of chaotic dendritic and axonic growth, with most of the resulting connections destined to disappear. But over subsequent decades the prevailing concept among neurobiologists and behavioral biologists was that synaptic connections increase with learning. Peter then rigorously showed in 1979 that after birth and an initial burst of growth in synapse numbers in human infants, there is a regression. He and his collaborators went on to show that these connections disappear at different times, with different kinetics, in distinct regions of the brain. The physical housekeeping task of this process is not small – selecting and eliminating billions of inactive synapses in the developing brain. In some regions of the brain, such as the visual system, the clearance mechanism seems to be relatively rapid over weeks or months. In other regions of the brain, for example in areas of higher cognitive function like the frontal cortex, this process of elimination is apparently more prolonged. What process or system has the intrinsic ability to identify and clear unused synapses? What has the ability to do this in a refined way, by targeting the correct contact sites, and without leaving dead cells and debris behind?

Phagocytes are a type of white blood cell that are in essence the vacuum cleaners of the body – sometimes known as the "professional eaters." Phagocytes eat cellular debris, dead cells and pathogens by engulfing their targets and degrading the debris in specialized intracellular compartments known as the lysosomes. Neutrophils and macrophages are the classic phagocytes, the primary cells of the innate immune system. Neutrophils are fast cells, specialized to remove foreign microbes, but after clearing microbes neutrophils can leave some damage in their midst. This is in contrast tomacrophages, roaming cells that play a surveillance role in tissues. Macrophages move through tissues slowly and work in a more refined manner by targeting debris or microbes using long thin projections, not unlike axons in morphology. Indeed, macrophages clear away neutrophils after neutrophils kill microbes, and limit tissue damage that neutrophils can leave behind. Together, these phagocytes collaborate to clean up and ward off disease. It is interesting that, in the brain, there are generally no neutrophils unless there is infection or abnormal inflammatory insult, as seen in neuroinflammatory disorders like multiple sclerosis. In the brain, there is a specialized type of macrophage, the microglial cell, that functions to clean up tissue damage and debris.

In the late 1800s, phagocytes were discovered by Elie Metchnikoff, the "father of immunology." Ramón y Cajal viewed neurons in preserved human brains, but Metchnikoff peered through microscopes at simple transparent sea organisms that were alive. In response to rose thorns or microbes, Metchnikoff watched in delight as he witnessed the "cellular act of eating." He named the cells "phagocytes," for cells (cytes) that eat (derived from the Greek word "phagein"). It is a dramatic process when phagocytes extend cell projections to engulf and devour microbes, foreign objects or cellular debris. Metchnikoff was a co-recipient of the 1908 Nobel Prize in Physiology or Medicine for this fundamental work.

At a phagocyte meeting in Sicily, where I first saw Professor Beth Stevens show the 1979 Peter Huttenlocher synaptic pruning slide, she was telling a beautiful story of her laboratory's work, uncovering how synapses in the developing brain are pruned. As her group worked on the visual circuits of mice, she discovered the unexpected. The brain phagocytes, the microglial cells, target and engulf synapses that are being eliminated. It makes sense that during a period of rapid regression in synapses, a phagocyte would be the engineer that makes it happen. During her postdoctoral work she had previously shown that the classic complement cascade mediates synapse elimination in the visual system of mice [1]. Complement proteins function in a cascade to activate the innate immune response to pathogens. They call for host defenses. In general, this response is proinflammatory and can contribute to tissue damage. Complement-mediated processes were generally known to be involved in pathologic responses to damage or infection, not normal developmental processes. Stevens' subsequent work showed that complement components tag synapses that are less active and ready for pruning. These tagged synapses are recognized by the complement receptor CR3 on microglial cells [2]. Their work demonstrated, for the first time, that pathogen-fighting complement proteins also mediate microglial synaptic pruning activity during normal development. Blocking these complement proteins impaired pruning in mouse models and altered the normal function of the visual circuits during development. This elegant work demonstrates that the complement system is critical for the normal developmental rewiring of brain circuitry that underlies the plasticity of the developing brain.

Related work on microglial cells was also going on in the laboratory of Cornelius Gross, but from a different perspective. With clear evidence that activity across synapses determines which ones are preserved or removed, Gross was also interested in what determines the structural remodeling of synaptic connections during development. His group observed the presence of synaptic material inside microglial cells, providing direct evidence that these cells can engulf synapses [3]. Gross focused on another small molecule, fractalkine, a chemokine that regulates phagocyte recruitment to damaged tissues. His group found that this small chemokine is expressed in synapses that are less active and, if you deplete it in mouse models, the circuitry of neurons in the brain is altered. His work provides further mechanisms for how microglial cells regulate synapse elimination.

Part of understanding a biological process is to identify the molecular players. The work of the Stevens and Gross laboratories places the complement system and fractalkine into the targeting piece of the puzzle. But in addition to having an on switch you need an off switch – the pathways that limit this irreversible change to brain circuitry. The Stevens laboratory identified a known pathway that protects from macrophage engulfment, a cell surface "cluster of differentiation" protein, CD47, that binds to the signal regulatory protein alpha (SIRPα) on macrophages and is known as a "don't eat me" signal. CD47 protects synapses from elimination. In mice deficient in CD47, the Stevens group found that there was increased microglial engulfment of synapses, and increased pruning [4]. Figure 17.1 summarizes some of the known pathways that positively and negatively regulate microglia-mediated synaptic pruning [5].

Despite this progress and glimpse of understanding, many challenges remain. In an interview with Beth Stevens in January 2022, she noted that "pruning is a permanent removal of synapses." The brain is adept at plasticity – the ability to change – to reform connections and edit out ones that are not needed. There are not just pruned synapses, but some connections are "weakened," like bad memories, and can erupt at later times. These types of "silent synapses" or weakened connections can be tapped and "called back into action." Another important concept is that some of the connections are inhibitory rather than excitatory, and a shift in the balance of excitatory and inhibitory connections can affect output. During development there are simply too many connections, and permanent changes to brain circuitry are needed to control this "cacophony" of signals. But, at later stages, these modifications in synapses may be more subtle, and not structural. The synapse may only become

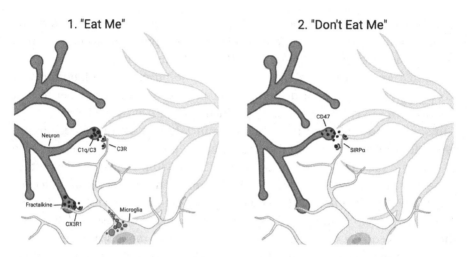

Figure 17.1 Schematic of microglial-cell-mediated synaptic pruning, showing the signals that mediate synapse removal by microglial cells ("eat me") including complement components C1q and C3 recognition by complement receptors on microglial cells and fractalkine–CX3R1 interactions. Microglial-cell-mediated pruning is inhibited by "don't eat me" signals mediated by CD47 and SIRPα. Figure by Alex Fister. Modeled after Rivest, 2018. Created with BioRender.com

quiescent rather than eliminated – and be available for future use when needed. It is likely that there is a continuum of modification, from elimination of synapses to their modification and, in essence, "turning off or on."

However, there is evidence that synaptic pruning, just like pruning a bush, occurs throughout life – and its aberrant activity can contribute to neurodegenerative diseases including Alzheimer's disease. Remarkably, work from Stevens and colleagues now has shown a genetic connection between complement protein expression and risk for Alzheimer's disease – with too much pruning and permanent removal of brain circuits later in life. In the case of Alzheimer's disease, distinct complement components have been implicated, including complement proteins C1q and C3, and this has implications for the treatment of Alzheimer's disease [6].

Stevens also commented on Feinberg's work and the hypothesis related to pruning and schizophrenia. "He leaned on Peter's data to back up this hypothesis and was inspired by him." Feinberg made the connection between sleep, adolescence and pruning. As Stevens noted:

When you sleep, what happens during sleep – active cognitive processes go offline – may be to make sure noncognitive things happen like lymphatic flux. "Sleep on it" – consolidating memories – strengthening them – the idea of "use it or lose it" – may occur in part at night. Maybe it is pruning of the connections that are not needed that occurs during sleep. Sleep and pruning.

And if sleep is disturbed, as it is in schizophrenia, this may contribute to abnormal pruning during adolescence and risk for schizophrenia.

Stevens went on to say that "immune system pruning is still a new concept," and much remains to be done to understand it. "Your dad inspired what we are doing. We do not know if schizophrenia and pruning is true, but now we have the tools to study it." The problem with this early work, and more recent studies, is that "it is a snapshot of a small region of the brain." It has been hard to repeat his work because of the difficulty getting fresh tissue and, because of the intrinsic variability of synapse number in different areas of brain tissue, there is a lot of "noise." To increase confidence in a finding you need to increase numbers of samples studied. There are plentiful data to support synaptic pruning in the sensory regions of the brain like the visual system – but there is a gap in understanding the frontal cortex, areas that control higher cognitive functions. Some of this gap can be addressed using animal models like mice or marmosets. Just as with Peter's work, "we have to understand the normal first in the frontal cortex of mammalian models – once you have the normal then you can study disease."

The idea that phagocytes and complement proteins have been repurposed in the brain for normal neurodevelopment is intriguing. The complement system, for example, is best known for its roles during infection and inflammation, but infection and inflammation can also affect the brain. "Neuroinflammation" arises when the immune systems of the brain – microglial cells, the complement system and other mediators – go into overdrive. This overdrive can contribute to the abnormal synaptic pruning and changes in brain circuitry recently noted in neuroinflammation. For example, in patients with the autoimmune disease systemic lupus erythematosis (lupus), neuroinflammation has recently been thought to be associated with abnormal pruning that can lead to neurological deficits. In addition, in the demyelinating autoimmune disease multiple sclerosis (MS), studies in both humans and mouse models have shown increased synapse loss in the visual system. A recent study reported increased C3 complement proteins at synapses in MS, and treatment with a complement inhibitor improved visual function in mouse models of MS [7]. In another example, Matt Johnson, a scientist at the Broad Institute at the Massachusetts Institute of Technology, studying synaptic pruning in Alzheimer's disease, said that the association of flu infection in pregnancy and the subsequent onset of schizophrenia may be related to neuroinflammation and pruning. In addition, the development of neuroinflammation around the time of birth is thought to disrupt synaptic pruning, potentially leading to neurodevelopmental disorders.

It is important to consider that microglial cells are likely not the whole story. Other cell types in the brain have been implicated in synaptic pruning, including the star-shaped astrocyte, the most abundant cell type in the human brain. Similar to microglial cells, astrocytes can engulf synapses in an activity-dependent manner. Indeed, mice that lack a key receptor for astrocyte engulfment, the multiple EGF-like-domains 10 (MEGF10), have impaired synaptic pruning in the visual system [8]. The astrocyte also releases factors that regulate microglial-cell-mediated pruning of synapses, suggesting that microglial cells and astrocytes likely collaborate to mediate the refined synaptic pruning necessary for normal development.

What is clear is that the next steps to understanding synaptic pruning in humans will require improved imaging. For example, imaging at the cellular level to determine if microglial cells directly eat synapses. The challenge remains that synapses are tiny and beyond the resolution of most light microscopes. Super-resolution imaging and three-dimensional reconstruction are needed to provide convincing evidence that synapses are inside microglial cells or in the lysosomal compartments of these cells that degrade debris. The possibility also exists that microglial cells act with more restraint, nibbling at synapses and altering their function. Could that contribute to a population of quiescent synapses that later are re-energized by activity of these quiescent connections? In addition to improved imaging of the cellular events, in humans, improved imaging of brain connectivity over time is needed. The advent of PET imaging to look at synapses in live human brains is a first step in this direction. But, in addition to imaging, analysis of human samples over time – like the levels of complement proteins in the cerebrospinal fluid that bathes the brain, may provide biomarkers to determine the extent of damage in disease states like schizophrenia or Alzheimer's disease. The ultimate goal for this work is to target specific pathways, such as particular complement constituents, to treat schizophrenia and Alzheimer's disease before the disease has irrevocably progressed. Some of these kinds of studies are in the works.

References

1. B. Stevens, N.J. Allen, L.E. Vazquez et al. The classical component cascade mediates CNS synapse elimination. *Cell* 2007; **131**: 1164–78.
2. D. P Schafer, E. K. Lehrman, A. G. Kautzman et al. Microglia sculpt postnatal neural circuits in an activity and complement-dependent manner. *Neuron* 2012; **74**: 691–705.

3. R. C. Paolicelli, G. Bolasco, F. Pagani et al. Synaptic pruning by microglia is necessary for normal brain development. *Science* 2011; **333**: 1456–8.

4. E. K. Lehrman, D. K. Wilton, E. Y. Litvina et al. CD47 protects synapses from excess microglia-mediated pruning during development. *Neuron* 2018; **100**: 120–34.

5. S. Rivest. A don't eat me immune signal protects neuronal connections. *Nature* 2018; **563**: 42–3.

6. S. Hong, VF Beja-Glasser, B.M. Nfonoyim et al. Complement and microglia mediate early synapse loss in Alzheimer mouse models. *Science* 2016; **352**: 712–16.

7. S. Werneburg, J. Jung, R. B. Kunjamma et al. Targeted complement inhibition at synapses prevents microglial synaptic engulfment and synapse loss in demyelinating disease. *Immunity* 2020; **52**: 167–82.

8. W. S. Chung, L. E. Clarke, G. X. Wang et al. Astrocytes mediate synapse elimination through MEGF10 and MERTK pathways. *Nature* 2013; **504**: 394–400.

18 LOOKING FORWARD: BEING A PHYSICIAN AND A SCIENTIST

The energy of the mind is the essence of life.
Aristotle, Greek philosopher (384–322 BCE)

Peter Huttenlocher was unendingly interested. Interested in music. In baking. In medicine. In people and their ways of thinking. In his patients. In the science of the human brain. "Peter is a great dreamer," said Hanne, Peter's paternal grandmother, in 1948. Although he delved deeply into philosophy in college, Peter decided early after arriving in the United States that he wanted to become a physician. He wanted to take care of people. So, he immersed himself in human medicine. He memorized. He took part in the multi-year training process for doctors that "knocks every ounce of originality out of you" [1].

Medicine requires certainty. It values decisiveness and a type of conformity. A respect for hierarchy and established protocol. Even as Peter delved into medical physiology, pathology, anatomy (and the grueling task of memorizing every muscle of the human body – over 600!), he also tried out science for the first time as a medical student. Science, unlike medicine, is uncertain and curiosity-driven. It requires a kind of wonderment as well as a measured disregard for authority and procedure. As a physician speaking to a patient, one is not supposed to say "I don't know." But for a scientist, "I don't know" is the start of the next question, the next experiment, the new frontier [2].

How does a physician scientist wed these conflicting styles? Why train in both science and medicine? Can't this merging of ideas and established knowledge be done efficiently by having scientists and physicians talk to each other? Absolutely – such collaboration is the backbone of biomedical science. However, the physician scientist is a different beast. There is something unique about understanding both the science and the medicine. For example, new connections between ideas are made when you walk into a patient's room. And if it is part of your job designation, the physician scientist (who is only a subset of the physicians even at a medical school) is enabled to "think outside the box" with a patient and take some risk. For example, develop a new ketogenic diet as a treatment for particularly problematic cases of epilepsy.

Physician scientists have often played a critical role in fundamental discoveries. An example is the discovery of statins – a medication that more than 35 million Americans in any given year take to lower their cholesterol and prevent heart disease. In the 1970s,Joseph Goldstein and Michael Brown, physician scientists at University of Texas Southwestern (UTSW), were intrigued by a group of patients at increased risk for cardiovascular disease who had an inherited form of high cholesterol, known as familial hypercholesterolemia. Brown and Goldstein discovered that patients with familial hypercholesterolemia lack a critical lipid receptor known as the low-density lipoprotein (LDL) receptor, resulting in high levels of the "bad" lipid, LDL, which is associated with heart disease. This work was recognized by the Nobel Prize in Physiology or Medicine in 1985. Brown and Goldstein and others went on to find that statins lower cholesterol in patients with high cholesterol, who are at risk for cardiovascular disease. This is a classic example of physician scientists going from the patient's "bedside" to the laboratory bench and back to the bedside with new knowledge that helps to advance new treatments.

The rare patient with a puzzling constellation of symptoms often finds their way into the physician scientist's clinic. Their disease may become the physician scientist's next experiment.Dan Kastner, a physician scientist at the National Institutes of Health (NIH), was puzzled by a group of patients with intermittent fevers, pain and systemic inflammation. Many of these patients have bizarre episodic symptoms that are debilitating, like patients with a disease called familial Mediterranean fever (FMF). Kastner and his colleagues uncovered the molecular defect in a protein, known as pyrin, that mediates FMF, launching a new set of discoveries that identified mechanisms for a group of disorders known as autoinflammatory diseases. Patients with these disorders have aberrant activation of inflammatory mediators known as cytokines, including interleukin 1 beta (IL1β). Kastner and others by now have identified many different autoinflammatory diseases in which cytokines are key, have advanced the field of immunology and have identified a key protein cluster known as the inflammasome that regulates IL1β activity. This work led to targeted therapies for autoinflammatory diseases through the inhibition of IL1β signaling (drugs such as anakinra). Treatment can be highly effective for patients with autoinflammatory diseases and other forms of systemic inflammation, including even cardiovascular disease. This is another example where physician scientists went from a rare disease to identifying mechanism to treatment. This work takes the collaboration of many scientists, physicians and physician scientists to finally reach the clinic and influence patient care. However, a key step along the way was the role of a physician scientist, Dan Kastner, who saw the patients and made pathbreaking connections regarding the disease mechanism and possible treatments.

Not all discoveries are worked out so quickly. Sometimes a discovery is made multiple decades before the development of associated disease treatments. This was the case with synaptic pruning. However, the fact that Peter had training in both medicine and science expedited the discovery. A non-clinician may have been less likely to even be studying post-mortem human brain specimens. A non-scientist might not have systematically counted synapses in multiple specimens. Peter's understanding of the human brain and the ways it goes wrong provided a perspective, helping him to know that what he was finding in his studies of those brain samples was startling. We noted above that, as a scientist, when one sees something potentially exciting, a standard reaction is to think "it cannot be true." But Peter figured out that what he was seeing was something fundamental that also explained much about the patients he saw in his clinic. Rather than ignore the oddities and pursue a different angle, he instead delved deeper.

Given the key insights and investigations so often launched by people with dual training in science and medicine, why is there a shortage of physician scientists? There has been much written about the "vanishing physician scientist" [3]. It is hard to do both science and medicine well, especially in the age of clinical productivity metrics where there is pressure to see more patients due to reimbursement schemes. It is hard to win competitive research grant funding when you are only doing science part-time. And it is hard, while hearing one's college friends speak of their new high-paying jobs and house purchases, to delay by multiple years one's rise out of lower-paying medical trainee positions and then earn less because of lower clinical throughput. It has pushed many physician scientists to make a choice between science and medicine, and to make the choice earlier in their career paths. This attrition of physician scientists is well documented and many solutions have been proposed. One key aspect of dual training – whether through a combined MD/PhD program or through later training of MDs after residency as research fellows – is to teach a willingness to, in essence, "dabble" and take some risks. We have seen that one driver of fundamental medical discoveries is a willingness to respond to the disparate patients that arrive through the door and dig deeply into what is going on. To think about the problem with a "curiosity." And to capitalize on that immense personal knowledge physician scientists possess of the human organism, spanning medicine and science. This is what drove Bill Kaelin, a physician scientist and cancer biologist who discovered a critical cancer pathway involving how cells sense and adapt to oxygen. He and a group of physician scientists, Peter Ratcliffe and Gregg Semenza, won the 2019 Nobel Prize in Medicine or Physiology for work that was influenced by the clinic and led to groundbreaking basic science discovery in oxygen sensing.

In part, this kind of thinking can be enabled by changes in medical education that encourage thinking out of the box, for both physicians and scientists. Training in fundamental research – allowing young physicians-to-be to receive the equivalent of a PhD in basic research – is critical for a subset of trainees. An additional element is to provide explicit training – role modeling – in translating findings from basic research to the clinic. A course developed as part of the University of Wisconsin–Madison MD/PhD program addresses this gap (other medical schools are also moving in this direction). In the final year of clinical training all dual-degree students engage in a clinical and translational research rotation, where they work closely with a physician scientist and develop a new translational research project that addresses a gap in patient treatment [4]. The class provides modeling of a physician scientist's career and also results in a translational research publication for many of the participants. Stated course goals are to train students to have a willingness to take risks, to immerse themselves in a new area inspired by patients and to integrate science and medicine.

It was this kind of focused "dabbling" that enabled Peter Huttenlocher's discovery of synaptic pruning. Major discoveries often start with an unexpected result. It can be a challenge to recognize the importance of the unexpected, especially if it is met with skepticism. This is where persistence and resilience come into play, traits that Peter certainly had learned during his childhood in Germany and as a new immigrant in the United States. Rejection is part of being a scientist (although rare for a doctor!). Perhaps more transparent persistence training will also be built into future physician scientist training curricula.

A productive population of physician scientists does not endure if the members are not also supported deep into their careers. MD/PhD training programs and early-career funding mechanisms, such as NIH K08 awards, launch many careers. But as with many other important findings, synaptic pruning was first described by a physician scientist who was between his late 40s and early 60s; an individual with many other demands on his time, who sustained the work through gaps in research funding. The support given to physician scientists at medical schools typically includes reduced clinical loads, provision of expensive laboratory space and well-placed internal funding. The money and space are borrowed from – prioritized over – other possible uses. This model has been successful: beneficial to the medical school's reputation and immensely beneficial to society at large. In the United States, financing for this system relies heavily on the overhead charged to research funding (for every $100,000 in funding that goes to a researcher, their university will typically collect an additional $50,000 to $70,000). But physician scientist support also draws from the larger pool of clinical revenue, and is constantly threatened by medical reimbursement schemes and accounting models that punish "inefficient" sectors. Mid- to late-career physician scientists are not likely to "vanish," but support for their explorations only continues when it is explicitly prioritized and battled for.

Once new biomedical science connections are made and an unexpected result becomes accepted, it becomes the work of many types of scientists to take the findings to the next level. The community digs deeper to understand the molecular mechanisms and practical utilities behind a process like synaptic pruning. In some ways, decades after the discovery of synaptic pruning, work in this field is just beginning. Questions are being generated more rapidly than answers, across a wide swath of applications from childhood learning to autism to psychiatric diseases and neurodegenerative diseases. It is not a simple gene disorder that leads to these aberrant conditions. Even within synaptic elimination, multiple pathways and mechanisms influence the refined process that is so central to human health. The initial discovery is now woven into the work of an incredibly diverse community of experts. This work is being supported because of its societal benefit – but a key part of it came into being in a setting where a conducive career path, persistent determination and financial support were available to a physician scientist.

References

1. C. M. Harper. Philosophy for physicians. *J R Soc Med* 2003; **96**: 40–5.
2. R. Lane. The widening chasm between research and clinical practice. *Sci Am* 0 2018; Nov 3.
3. A. I. Schafer. The vanishing physician scientist? *Transl Res* 2010; **155**: 1–2.
4. J. Stefely, E. Theisen, C. Hanewall et al. A physician-scientist preceptorship in clincal and translational research enhances training and mentorship. *BMC Med Educ* 2019; **19**: 89.

19 PARKINSON'S DISEASE AND BERLIN

In the summer of 2012, Peter said to me: "I have become an expert on Parkinson's dementia." He paused with a smile, his quiet humor intact after more than two decades of Parkinson's disease. His next sentence came out after a bit of effort. "It is all about the synapses and abnormal pruning."

Peter was 60 years old in 1991 when he was diagnosed with Parkinson's disease. When I was a medical student home on holiday, I noticed a change in his gait and asked, "Dad: do you think you have Parkinson's disease?" He replied, "Yes. I am worried about that." For years after that, Peter was under clinical care for Parkinson's. The treatment primarily consisted of lifestyle changes and as little L-dopamine as possible to control his symptoms. He did well for the first decade or more after diagnosis. He continued seeing patients, socializing, attending events and traveling. As the years passed, in the second decade after diagnosis, Peter needed to increase the medicine to control his symptoms and compensate for the low levels of the neurotransmitter dopamine that is characteristic of Parkinson's. The progression of the disease is often gradual, over years. Peter had been an avid hiker, with a long and fast stride. His gait visibly declined over these years, at first changing to smaller, slower steps, and later to the shuffling gait of Parkinson's disease.

Parkinson's disease's progression is gradual, but insidious. The voice diminishes and muscles become more rigid. Facial expressions, and seemingly emotions, fade. Movement becomes difficult and tremors become common. Mental status starts to wax and wane. The social network for people with Parkinson's disease narrows. For Peter as well, less and less time was spent interacting with friends, and he spent more time with his family (Figure 19.1).

In 2003, after Peter retired from the University of Chicago, Janellen was invited to spend a year as a fellow at the Wissenschaftskolleg, an interdisciplinary institute in the western part of Berlin. Wissenschaftkolleg brings together scientists from around the world, to discuss work in the social and natural sciences. Peter was interested in living in Germany for the year. Until his father passed away around 1990, he had enjoyed almost yearly visits to Europe for work and to see his father and brothers in Munich. He particularly enjoyed visits to his father.

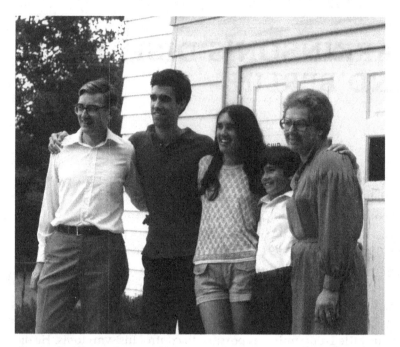

Figure 19.1 Photo of Peter with his family in 1984.

As Janellen later said, "Richard enjoyed good conversation." An earlier family letter said, "Opa Huttenlocher is really quite a card – constantly coming up with funny lines but also dead set in his own ideas. Somehow, Wolfie [Wolfgang] and I got to discussing atomic power and Opa could not tolerate any opinion other than his own which is pro-Nuke." Peter saved the many letters that Richard sent to him over the years. He was proud of his father's many patents and that he started a chemistry journal, *Tensid* (now known as *Tenside Surfactants and Detergents*). On a recent visit to Munich's Englischer Garten with Wolfgang, we walked to the Bogenhausen neighborhood and passed the Carl Hanser Verlag building, home to the publishing company where Richard worked on the *Tensid* journal. This was close to the Thomas Mann house in Munich, a villa on a quiet tree-lined street in Bogenhausen. Thomas Mann, the winner of the Nobel Prize in Literature in 1929 and author of *The Magic Mountain*, fled Germany in 1933. He wrote political works that criticized the Nazi regime and were banned by the government. He also publicly declared his support for German writers who had been exiled by the German government. Like Peter's mother, Thomas Mann's citizenship was rescinded and he was banned from working in Germany. He moved to Switzerland and then to the United States. Peter had previously shared stories that, during the war, Richard, Dieter and Peter listened to Mann's anti-

Nazi speeches that were broadcast by the BBC on the long-wave radio to Germany.

Many years had passed since Richard's death when Janellen received the invitation to work in Berlin, but Peter welcomed a year in Europe in the twilight of his career. Living again in Germany provided thought-provoking stimulation, some more welcome and some less so, especially with the challenges of Parkinson's disease. He relished the opportunity to see the Munich family and to visit places from his childhood. Peter's brothers Wolfgang and Götz visited him in Berlin, and his US family also visited. During this time, Peter's health rallied and he seemed to effortlessly hop on and off buses during exploratory trips around Berlin. The rich, lush western regions of Berlin and the Brandenburg Gate stood in contrast to the former East Berlin, still stark but with a raw and lively young energy.

During the year in Berlin, one journey was to his childhood home in Braubach with his wife, daughter and grandchildren. The trip took a diversion to Harburg, a medieval village with a castle and many small farms. Peter's family friends farmed in Harburg and, for a few summers, young Peter had gone alone by train to work on their farm. Peter described the summers on the farm: he traveled loaded with a suitcase full of soap from his father's chemical company, which he would offer in exchange for meat – pork – from the farm. He worked for several weeks on the farm to further cover the cost (and perhaps to keep him productively busy). Farms were short of help at the time and Peter was a hard worker. On the train route back home, the luggage would be heavy with meat, but Peter pretended the luggage was light as he quickly walked past guards, avoiding the guard dogs in particular. It was against the law to transport meat since food was being rationed and meat was prioritized for soldiers. It was strategic to have a young boy transport the meat because he was less likely to arouse suspicion or to be punished if he was discovered.

As Peter and his family drove in 2003 across a bridge into the town of Harburg and turned on a bend in the road, Peter exclaimed: "That is where the barn was that housed the pigs!" The "barn" site was now a government bureau with computers and workers. But the old farmhouse was still intact and clearly continued to be used as a residence. Without advance notice Peter knocked on the door and, sure enough, Annie, the farmer's daughter, a few years older than Peter, answered. She looked and examined him for a moment standing on her doorstep. They quickly recognized each other despite the elapsed years and she exclaimed "Peter!" in delight. She served tea and German kuchen as if she had been preparing for the visit. The conversation quickly turned to the war. Her family was anti-Nazi but that had become untenable for her father. He had to join the party late in the war to sell his

grain, and the Nazis confiscated their meat. She lamented that many of the
Nazis in town later became the town leaders after the war but people in town
did not speak about the war. At the end of the war, the Nazis had bombed the
old bridge into town to try to stop the Allied forces. As Annie said: "even if all of
the women and children in town were on the bridge, the German soldiers
would have bombed it." The 70-plus-year-old Annie was sprightly and showed
Peter around the remaining farm buildings. Peter and Annie looked at each
other sadly and hugged before departing.

It was during the year in Berlin that Janellen first noticed some cognitive
decline with Peter. Parkinson's disease can be associated with both early cognitive dysfunction and later dementia. Janellen raised concerns about cognitive
decline in a family email during their time at the Wissenshaftkolleg, 13 years
after his diagnosis of Parkinson's disease. First in jest, Peter and Janellen wrote:

> Hi,
>
> I hope you answer your email. I am afraid that we thought the phone was
> the doorbell. We are yoyos. A colleague was here and pointed out the
> problem. We should have because no one was ever at the door. Hiccup.
>
> > Love,
> > Mom and Dad

Then a more serious email from Janellen:

> Hi,
>
> You know I didn't respond to you last night in terms of what I have been
> thinking. As you know, Parkinson's slows down all processes. There is con-
> siderable recent work in psychology showing this effect in memory – slowing
> down in search processes. It is my idea that this is Dad's problem. Whenever
> he sets his mind to a problem he is as sharp as ever. I notice that when he is
> distracted like with the wonderful presence of his daughter and grandchil-
> dren, wonderful new things like concerts, that is when the system sort of
> "blows." I am trying to think of ways to make him realize that he will find
> whatever information it is that he cannot find "on-line" fast and make him
> look less bewildered and out of it. He always had a slight tendency that way
> anyhow. So, your cognitive psychologist mom is trying to think out how to
> help him cope. But I do believe the problem is isolated this way. Do you think
> this is a possible interpretation?
>
> > All my love,
> > Mom

After their return to the United States, Janellen spent the subsequent years helping Peter (and herself) cope with progressing Parkinson's disease, especially by keeping active. She organized attendance at concerts and plays, dinners out with friends and travel to visit family. After their return from Berlin, Peter needed more help. He selected a Polish immigrant as his caregiver. Josef was an incredibly kind man, with some language gaps but with a shared interest and advanced knowledge of classical music. Together, Peter, Janellen and Josef attended many concerts and traveled for family visits.

On Peter's final trip to Europe at the age of 80, Peter and Janellen visited family when they were on sabbatical in Basel, Switzerland. The extended family had a reunion in the Swiss mountains, which included Peter's brother Wolfgang. One afternoon, Wolfgang and Peter decided the two of them would take a drive and Janellen reluctantly agreed, reluctant because she was concerned about Peter and trusted neither Wolfgang's fast driving nor his judgment with Peter. Janellen displayed increasing angst when, after many hours, the brothers still failed to return. Then, as evening descended, Wolfgang and Peter arrived in Wolfgang's sports car – with big smiles. They had driven through the mountains, stopped at a few cafes, and spontaneously taken a boat trip across the lake. Peter looked mischievously happy. Quiet and pleased. Wolfgang looked like a scolded schoolboy, but also thrilled to have taken his older brother, with advanced Parkinson's disease, on such an adventure.

Even with advancing Parkinson's disease, Peter continued to ponder synaptic pruning and its implications. When musing that he had become a first-hand expert on Parkinson's dementia ("it is all about synaptic pruning"), he may have hit upon something. Parkinson's disease is most associated with a loss of neurons in the midbrain basal ganglia structure known as the substantia nigra and the associated loss of dopamine production. The dementia is associated with the presence of cortical and subcortical alpha-synuclein/Lewy bodies, but postmortem studies of patients with Parkinson's disease dementia often reveal the co-existence of pathologies associated with Alzheimer's disease. Recent findings (discussed in a previous chapter) suggest that microglial cells and abnormal synaptic pruning may be implicated in Alzheimer's disease. Is Parkinson's disease dementia also mediated in part by aberrant synaptic pruning? Recent evidence suggests that this may be the case.

20 AUF DEUTSCH: BACK TO GERMAN

Schön ist es auch anderswo, und hier bin ich sowieso.

(It is beautiful elsewhere, and here I am anyways.)

Wilhelm Busch, German poet (1832–1908)

Ich bin müde.

(I am tired.)

Peter Huttenlocher

In the later stages of Parkinson's disease most patients develop progressive cognitive impairment and dementia. During his final year, Peter often spoke in German. He alternated between disorientation and lucidity. During his disoriented periods, he wandered. At night he would scream out in terror. It became clear that he needed round-the-clock care and, after much hesitation, his family all decided that he needed to live in the care facility connected to Peter and Janellen's retirement community. The iron grip of Parkinson's disease is difficult for families. It is a confusing kind of dementia, the periods of lucidity raising hopes that are repeatedly dashed. Peter was locked in during those last months. It was not always clear he recognized his friends or family members, but sometimes he made so much sense! "Ich bin müde" (I am tired) or "genug" (enough), he said.

On one of his lucid days in his final year of life, the family took him out of the care facility and gathered at the cottage near Lake Michigan where Janellen and Peter had spent weekends since moving to Chicago. When cleaning out his desk the family discovered a box of letters written between family members during and after the war. Some of these letters were written by Peter and told stories about food and the garden. Some were thank-you notes for Christmas packages from Else to the four boys with chocolate and gifts from the United States. Peter had never told his family about the letters. Curious, his family started to ask more questions. Peter spoke and told stories he had not told before.

He spoke about his mother, Else. "She did not have to leave." Startled, we asked: "What do you mean?" Peter replied: "If she had been quiet, she could have stayed." He had always talked proudly about his mother speaking out against Nazism. But it now appeared that this pride had always served as a mask for the little boy wishing for his mother. We spoke about his mother: about hiking in the Adirondacks with his mother in the years after Peter's arrival in the United States, and about annual family visits to East Eden, in the farmland of western New York State. During those summers Else's grandchildren ran amok in the fields, and along "Peter's path" in the forest behind the house. They climbed into the tree house or scrambled up rocky cliffs, went swimming in the local swimming hole. At night, Else banished the grandchildren to the summer cottage to sleep (the children were also banished for an hour in the afternoon every day so that Oma and Opa could watch their beloved soap opera, *The Guiding Light*, about "the Bauers," a middle-class German immigrant family). Else, endearingly called Moo Coo by Peter and Dieter, loved to cook German feasts of *spätzle* and *sauerbraten*. Else would sit in the yard feeding the hummingbirds from her hand. She raised an abandoned nest of baby robins, and they (or their relations) returned each summer – also to be fed from Oma's hand. Else died unexpectedly in her sleep in 1970, of a hypertensive stroke, at 66 years of age. A death that with medical advances, is preventable, it shocked the family. Peter and Dieter had 20 years with their mother in the United States. But it was not long enough. As Peter said, "She did not have to leave." She had fled again, without her children.

Toward the end of Dieter's life, Dieter also spoke about his childhood in ways his family had not heard. He told the horrifying tale from before Else fled, about the public execution of the mayor and townspeople who spoke out against the treatment of the nearby Jewish community. As it turns out, five-year-old Peter, accompanied by his eight-year-old brother Dieter, happened to be wandering through the town center together one day and witnessed one of these hangings. Dieter quickly escorted his younger brother out of the town center, back toward their home. They never spoke about it. It was shortly after this episode that Else left Germany for Belgium, never returning, and Richard moved with the boys to Greiz in the east of Germany. It was not safe for any of them to remain in their village along the Rhine. Richard approached the Nazi regime with silent dissent and his children also lived through the war in silent dissent. The guilt and shame of having lived through this, even as children, was something that haunted their final days.

Before Peter and Dieter departed Germany, Richard had written to Else: "Let the boys find their peace – and let them find their way to separate themselves from their past." Peter and Dieter moved forward but in different ways. Peter set forth on his path with quiet stoicism, avoiding conflict or attention. Dieter moved forward first with rage (for example, he smashed his step-father's lawn mower with a sledge hammer shortly after arriving in the United States). But later Dieter centered himself with his outgoing and jovial humor and successful work as a chemical engineer. He was loud and fun, while Peter was a dreamer and more quiet. Although different in personality, Dieter and Peter remained very close. In his confusion in the final year, Peter would often call out for his brother Dieter, who had passed away the year before. Like Peter, in the final months of his life, Dieter experienced depression and disturbing childhood memories. Dieter had advanced heart disease and stopped eating in the final months of his life, gradually fading to 105 pounds. Dieter had only returned to Germany once as an adult, to attend his 50th high-school reunion in Greiz. Of his classmates, two had gone to America, and ten had died in French war camps.

As we have heard, Peter was a *Kriegskind*, a war child. He was too young for direct participation in the war, but old enough to remember the bombs, the hunger, the separation from his mother and then father, and the fear. He also experienced the feelings of guilt and shame, during the war, after the war and as a German immigrant in the United States. Was this the sadness that seemed to amplify in the later years of his life?

21 MEMORIES AND REFLECTIONS AT THE END: A RETURN TRIP TO GREIZ

Let them forget the war years in Greiz.

Richard Huttenlocher

Peter returned to Greiz only once, in 1990 with his family, 44 years after he escaped from the Soviet zone with his stepmother and brothers. On this visit to the home of his childhood memories, the Berlin wall had just fallen but the German reunification was yet to come. East Germany – the German Democratic Republic – had existed as a nation since 1949, having transitioned from being a Soviet-occupied zone to statehood, but of course remaining under heavy Soviet influence. Peter's visit was to an East Germany that was gradually being disbanded. It was still a communist nation, but citizens of the German Democratic Republic could now travel abroad. Through the centralized East German government, Peter had arranged modest accommodations in the old - town area of Greiz, where no direct bookings or modern hotels existed at that time.

I took part in that trip with my husband, mother and young son. On arrival to East Germany, we passed through border patrol with our travel papers in order. But the East German border guards looked disinterested and did not check passports. These were two separate countries, but everyone knew that would not last much longer. The villages of East Germany stood in striking contrast to the villages in the neighboring West. There were buildings in ruins, and modest little dark and old cars. The "Eastern-style" drab apartment buildings, largely concrete, seemed to have been erected with speed and without consideration for architectural style. However, the old town of Greiz was still picturesque and had largely avoided being destroyed during the war. As we walked through the old town, we were charmed. Charmed until we passed a small square and Peter grimly pointed to it as the spot where, in the final years of the war, young army deserters had been publicly hanged as an example. We moved on.

The old family house, where Peter's family had rented an apartment, was in a hillside neighborhood that overlooked the town, with rolling hills and open fields nearby. Peter's mood had picked up and the memories – bits and snip-pets – were flowing. The garage, which had been bombed, had been replaced with something new, cement and practical, but the house otherwise looked just like he remembered. Peter thought it might be possible to get a peek inside. We were met with suspicion and a distinctly unfriendly greeting from a woman who lived there. Peter explained that this had been his childhood home, and asked if he could just show it to his wife, daughter and grandson. Further soured, she refused our entry.

Upon arrival to our rooming house, we were greeted by a gruff older woman who spoke with the rough local accent and was not eager to help. She said: "I have no record of a booking." Peter responded, *auf Deutsch* (in German): "We booked it officially through the East German government." There was "no record." Peter and the woman went back and forth for multiple minutes, Peter ending with: "We will not leave until you have found us a place to stay." There were no other nearby options, Peter's two-year-old grandson was tired and getting fussy and Peter's Germanic confidence was strong because he had followed proper procedures and had paperwork showing booked rooms for his family. After an extended debate, they found a room of sorts. The laundry room was temporarily equipped with four portable beds and a crib. Interestingly, the younger employees were curious and eager to help, and cheerfully provided information about the few dining options in Greiz. Under further curious gazes from local residents, we enjoyed a perfectly acceptable meal.

The next day we took the ancient, wooden-benched but still functioning narrow-gauge train to Neumühle, through the forests near Greiz (Figure 21.1). Peter was particularly eager to take his grandson on the old trains of his childhood – the same train cars that had been in operation decades before. We hiked in the woods near Neumühle, where, as a child, he had pushed a wheelbarrow in search of food and provisions for his family. The return visit to Greiz was brief, but it was during this visit Peter spoke freely for the first time about his some of his memories from the war. Memories that had long been suppressed.

He did not tell all of the painful stories about Greiz during that visit. It is unclear if some of these were suppressed memories or if he did not want to talk about them. In the last year of his life, on that afternoon in Michigan, Peter first shared his memories of a particularly distressing experience in Greiz. With a look of terror in his eyes Peter said:

When I was 14 years old, 1945, I was late to school, as I often was. It was a long walk, and I lacked motivation. When I arrived at the schoolhouse, with 40

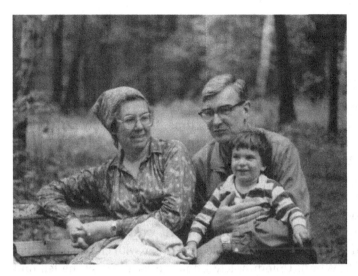

Figure 21.1 Peter with his grandson and Janellen in the woods in Neumühle, near Greiz, in 1990. Peter had roamed these woods, as a child, looking for food during the war.

students, it was shortly after a bomb had hit. The bomb destroyed the school, it was in ruins. Some of my schoolmates and teachers were killed. I saw one of my classmates, dead, near the entrance of the school. I was alive because I was a poor student. Because I was late.

Other family members later verified the bombing, although it was the first time Peter had spoken to any of his children about it.

It is hard to comprehend how a young child witnesses such devastation and moves forward. There is substantial recent research on the inhibitory networks in the brain that suppress these unwanted memories [1]. Apparently, forgetting is an active process that is mediated by inhibitory control mechanisms in the brain that stop painful memories. It is referred to as motivated forgetting. The inhibitory control mechanisms are in the frontal lobe of the brain. Evidence suggests that the neurotransmitter dopamine can affect these inhibitory networks in the prefrontal cortex to promote adaptive forgetting [2]. Dopamine is deficient in patients with Parkinson's disease. It is intriguing to speculate that this may have contributed to what happened with Peter in his final year of life, with the night screams and resurfacing of painful memories. Researchers are making strides in understanding how unwanted memories are suppressed, although the area is still in its infancy. Do Parkinson's patients have re-emergence of these thoughts due to the loss of dopamine activity in these inhibitory networks? Or is it possible that these inhibitory networks and synapses are pruned aberrantly in Parkinson's disease and this contributes to the unleashing of repressed memories later in the disease?

The Final Months

In the final months of Peter's life, in the lucid moments, he spoke more often about his childhood in Germany. But at other times he spoke only in German. It was often difficult to understand. English and German were mixed together. We would often sing German songs with him – we would sing the classic Brahms lullaby "Guten Abend, Gute Nacht" (good evening, goodnight) – he sang it perfectly, and looked subdued, even happy.

During one of the visits in his final months he kept trying to stand, but he was not allowed to stand because he had been falling. He was strong and stubborn. I would say "Sitzen" (Sit down) and he would look at me with childlike mischief and say "Warum?" (Why?). Unfortunately, shortly after this visit, he fell and broke his hip. I spoke with his nurse on the phone, and she told me he was in severe pain. I visited to check on him. With any movement he would cry out in agonizing pain, but the physician in the care center had no plans to fix his hip. This unshaven and "demented" old man, who had been fluent in English, was now speaking in German and people could not understand him. It was assumed that he was too far gone to worry about his pain. I was horrified that the care facility would leave him with a fractured hip. I called the local orthopedic surgeon and persuaded them to pin his hip. The local University of Chicago hospital was very nice about his care and allowed me to accompany him into the operating room and keep him calm as he was put to sleep. He did well during the procedure and spent the final six months of his life without hip pain. To this day I wonder if, without a strong advocate – a physician daughter – he would have been left with an untreated hip fracture and excruciating pain. It certainly did not matter that he had previously been a distinguished scientist and physician.

A few months later I wrote in my journal about another day's visit to Peter with my cousin, Dieter's daughter Gail:

When we arrived, dad no longer wore his glasses, and his brilliant blue-green eyes, like Dieter's, shined and softened with a warm smile when we entered the room. Gail cried when she saw him. While we were there he was pointing at a paper cup, and I handed it to him. He tried to drink from the cup. But it was empty. He was puzzled. I got him something to drink and helped him with it. Then he picked up the empty cup again, thinking it was full and tried to drink and was again puzzled when nothing came out. He put his hand in the cup and realized it was empty and laughed. Gail laughed, we all laughed.

On August 16, 2013, I wrote:

I am watching the sun rise over Lake Michigan from my parent's apartment. Reflections in the water. My dad died yesterday. 82 years old. I arrived the night before and sat with him. Rapid breathing but sleeping quietly with occasional twitching. He responded but did not seem aware. Last weekend he was very aware – more than the months before. It was difficult to speak – and he used all of his energy and with great effort, looked me in the eyes and said "I love you."

Yesterday morning rapid breathing, responsive to touch. I went for a walk along Lake Michigan, on the beach and sat on the rocks and then returned to his room. A change in his breathing had occurred during my absence and his nurse recommended that my mom come to his side. My mom and I were sitting with my dad. There were longer pauses in his breathing and he was peaceful. We held his hand.

Then our German friend Ruth joined us, and the minister, Father Petite. We sat and spoke about my dad and laughed. Sighs and gaps. I held his hand. Together we sang "Guten Abend, Gute Nacht." My dad opened his eyes and looked at us; peaceful, gave a big sigh, and he was gone. No more breathing. Quiet.

> Guten Abend, Gut Nacht.
> Mit Rosen bedacht.
> Mit Näglein besteckt.
> Shlupf unter die Deck.
> Morgen Früh, wenn Gott will
> Wirst du wieder geweckt.
> Morgen Früh wenn Gott will
> Wirst du wieder geweckt.
>
> Good evening, good night,
> With roses covered,
> With cloves adorned,
> Slip under the covers.
> Tomorrow morning, if God wills,
> you will wake once again
> Tomorrow morning, if God wills,
> you will wake once again.

At Peter's memorial service, Unitarian minister and good friend Donald Wheat ended the sermon by saying that Peter was lucky to have lived such a rich life, even though it had been bracketed by difficult years at the beginning and end. I pondered this. His life had been rich with experience and partnership and, most importantly, rich because of how he had lived it. It made me think about the words of the nineteenth-century American naturalist and philosopher Henry David Thoreau: "I went to the woods because I wished to live deliberately, to front only the essential facts of life, and see if I could not learn what it had to teach, and not, when I came to die, discover that I had not lived. I did not wish to live what was not life."

References

1. M. C. Anderson and S. Hanslmayr. Neural mechanisms of motivated forgetting. *Trends Cogn Sci* 2014; **18**: 279–92.
2. M. Wimber, B. H. Schott, F. Wendler et al. Prefrontal dopamine and the dynamic control of human long-term memory. *Transl Psychiatry* 2011; **1**: e15.

GLOSSARY

Actin: A family of proteins that form microfilaments in the cytoskeleton of the cell and also form fibrils in muscle cells. Actin polymerization is a critical process that is involved in cell movement.

Action potential: A large electrical current, lasting one to two milliseconds, which propagates along the axon's presynaptic terminal. At this terminal, electrical activity leads to the release of neurotransmitter onto the post-synaptic terminal of the target neuron.

Alzheimer's disease: A neurodegenerative disease that is progressive with age and is associated with dementia.

Aphasia: A group of language disorders that result from lesions in specific regions of the brain that control language. Different types of aphasia include Wernicke's aphasia or the ability to understand language and Broca's aphasia, the ability to speak.

Astrocyte: Star-shaped glial cells in the brain and spinal cord. They are the most plentiful cell type in the brain and play a critical supportive role in providing nutrients and other signals to the neurons.

Autism or autism spectrum disorder: A group of neurodevelopmental disorders generally with onset in childhood that influence how the affected individual interacts with others, learns and communicates.

Axon: The long extension that emanates from the cell body of the neuron and ends in presynaptic terminals, where it connects to other cells and sends signals.

Basal ganglia: A region of the brain that controls movement and is involved in Parkinson's disease. Neurons in the basal ganglia produce dopamine, the neurotransmitter that is deficient in Parkinson's disease.

Brain: A complex organ that mediates memory, emotion, movement, sensation and all behavior. It is made of different parts including the cerebrum, the cerebellum and the brain stem. The brain communicates to the body through the spinal cord.

Broca's area: A region of the brain in the left frontal cortex that is involved in spoken or written language.

Cell migration: The process by which cells move during development and the formation of multicellular organisms. This can involve the directed movement of single cells, like immune cells, or groups of cells.

Cerebral cortex: The outer region of the cerebral hemisphere, which is comprised of the frontal, parietal, temporal and occipital lobes.

Cerebral hemispheres: The two hemispheres of the brain, connected by axons referred to as the corpus callosum, which coordinate the activities of these two hemispheres. Each cerebral hemisphere is composed of the cortex, the basal ganglia (controls movement), hippocampus (memory) and amygdala (emotions like fear).

Cognition: The process of acquiring knowledge and understanding the senses, experience and thought. Cognitive psychology is focused on the study of mental processes. Cognitive neuroscience is the study of the brain.

Complement component: A plasma or blood protein that is comprised of many distinct components. The proteins work with the immune system to combat infection and activate both the innate (phagocytes) and adaptive (T cells) parts of the immune system. Genetic changes in specific complement component abnormalities (C3, C1q) have been associated as a risk factor for Alzheimer's disease and schizophrenia.

Cytoskeleton: A network of microscopic filaments and tubules in the cytoplasm of cells that give the cell its shape and regulate the ability of individual cells to migrate.

Dendrite: A branched extension that emanates from the cell body of a neuron and receives signals from other neurons through the synapse.

Dopamine: A neurotransmitter that controls voluntary movement and cognition. Deficiency of dopamine is found in Parkinson's disease. An excess of dopaminergic signaling has been implicated in schizophrenia.

Epilepsy: A disorder of the brain characterized by seizures or involuntary movements, due to electrical dysfunction of the brain.

Filamin: A group of large proteins that bind to the actin cytoskeleton and to adhesion receptors on the surface of cells. Filamins regulate cell adhesion and migration.

Fractalkine: A small protein or chemokine that mediates inflammation.

Frontal lobe: A lobe in the cerebral cortex that mediates executive functions like memory, speech and movement of the body.

Golgi stain: A silver staining technique that is used to image neurons using light microscopy.

Interneuron: A type of neuron that connects between neurons and regulates their activity. Some interneurons inhibit the activity of other neurons (inhibitory neurons).

Ketogenic diet: A low-carbohydrate, high-fat diet that is used to treat people with seizure disorders.

Lateral geniculate nucleus (LGN): A structure in the thalamus that is part of the mammalian visual pathway. It is in an area of thalamus that connects with the optic nerve.

Lysosome: An organelle within all cells that gets rid of the waste within the cell, a type of garbage can. It degrades material that is taken up by phagocytes, including cellular debris or pathogens.

Magnetic resonance imaging (MRI): A non-invasive imaging method that uses a magnet to image structures in the brain. Functional MRI is a method that uses MRI to detect changes in blood flow and oxygen consumption in the brain, to detect regions of the brain that are more or less active.

Memory: The encoding of data or information.

Microglial cell: A specialized type of phagocyte that is found in the brain and removes damaged cells and neurons and helps to control infection.

Motor neuron: A type of neuron that controls muscle and movement. Motor neurons make synapses with muscle cells sending information from the central nervous system (CNS) to control movement.

Nerve: A nerve is comprised of a bundle of axons that transmit information from neurons.

Neural circuit: A network that forms between a group of neurons that are interconnected and influence each other's activity.

Neurology: The area of medicine focused on the brain and how it goes awry in disease. Neurologists focus on the care of patients with diseases of the nervous system, including seizure disorders, stroke, Alzheimer's disease and Parkinson's disease.

Neuron: The primary cell of the nervous system. There are approximately 100 billion neurons in the human brain. Each neuron makes around 1,000 synapses, resulting in a complex network of connections. Neurons can extend long distances from the brain to the periphery with the cell body, often a meter or more away from some of the synapses that an individual neuron makes.

Neurotransmitter: A chemical released by an activated neuron that activates an adjacent cell (typically another neuron). It is a chemical that is released by one neuron through its synapse and binds to the receptor on another neuron, altering the flow of current in the receiving neuron.

Parkinson's disease: A neurological disorder associated with deficiency in brain cells in the basal ganglia that make dopamine. Parkinson's symptoms often develop gradually over years and include progressive movement disorders such as tremor, loss of balance and a shuffling gait as well as non-motor symptoms such as depression, anxiety, sleep disorders and various cognitive impairments.

Periventricular heterotopia: A rare neurological disease that commonly presents with seizures, and is associated with a defect in neuronal cell migration early in development.

Phagocyte: A type of innate immune cell in the body that can engulf and remove cellular debris and pathogens. The two primary cells of the innate immune system are neutrophils and macrophages. Microglial cells are a type of macrophage.

Plasticity: The ability of neurons and their connections (synapses) to change based on experience and activity.

Positron-emission tomography (PET): PET is a type of imaging method that reports brain function through the use of radioactive molecules to probe specific brain activities. This can be used to read out the metabolism or blood flow in the brain. More recent methods are used to quantify synapses in different regions of the brain (using the SV2A synapse marker).

Protein: A biomolecule made up of amino acids. Thousands of different proteins in any cell are enzymes that catalyze the chemical reactions of life, while other proteins can serve structural roles.

Reflex: An involuntary unlearned response to an external stimulus, like the knee jerk test, commonly done by neurologists. In the case of the spinal reflex like the knee jerk reflex, it is mediated by neurons in the spinal cord and does not require signals from the brain.

Rapid eye movement (REM): At night you fluctuate between two types of sleep, REM sleep and non-REM sleep. REM sleep is associated with rapid movement of eyes and increased brain activity during sleep. REM sleep is associated with dreaming and the consolidation of memories.

Rett syndrome: A rare genetic disorder that affects brain development in girls. It is a type of neurodevelopmental autism spectrum disorder.

Reye's syndrome: A rare, serious brain condition linked with aspirin use during viral infections in children, and associated with liver and brain damage.

Schizophrenia: A serious mental illness that affects how a person thinks, acts and feels.

Sensory neuron: One of the three major types of neurons. Sensory neurons detect sensation in the periphery like touch.

Synapse: The point of contact between two neurons through which signals and information are transmitted. The synaptic cleft is the gap between two neurons through which chemical signals are propagated.

Synaptogenesis: The developmental process of the formation of synapses, maintenance of synapses and activity-dependent elimination of synapses.

Systemic lupus erythematosus (lupus): A systemic autoimmune disease in which the immune system attacks its own tissues and leads to inflammation in multiple organs, including the joints, skin, brain and kidney.

Tuberous sclerosis: A rare genetic condition that causes benign tumors in different tissues, including the brain.

Visual system: A sensory circuit that travels from the retina of the eye to the cortex. This is the circuit that Hubel and Wiesel dissected to understand how vision works.

Wernicke's area: The region of the left parietal lobe that handles language comprehension.

INDEX